Nursing and the Division of Labour in Healthcare

Sociology and Nursing Practice Series

Davina Allen and David Hughes
Nursing and the Division of Labour in Healthcare

Lorraine Culley and Simon Dyson (editors)
Ethnicity and Nursing Practice

Margaret Miers
Gender Issues and Nursing Practice

Sam Porter
Social Theory and Nursing Practice

Geoff Wilkinson and Margaret Miers (editors)
Power and Nursing Practice

Sociology and Nursing Practice Series
Series Standing Order
ISBN 0–333–69329–9
(outside North America only)

You can receive future titles in this series as they are published by placing a standing order. Please contact your bookseller or, in the case of difficulty, write to us at the address below with your name and address, the title of the series and the ISBN quoted above.

Customer Services Department, Macmillan Distribution Ltd
Houndmills, Basingstoke, Hampshire RG21 6XS, England

Also by Davina Allen:
The Changing Shape of Nursing Practice: The Role of Nurses in the Hospital Division of Labour

Nursing and the Division of Labour in Healthcare

Davina Allen and David Hughes

with

Sue Jordan, Morag Prowse
and Sherrill Snelgrove

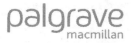

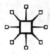
First published 2002 by
PALGRAVE MACMILLAN
Houndmills, Basingstoke, Hampshire RG21 6XS and
175 Fifth Avenue, New York, N.Y. 10010
Companies and representatives throughout the world

PALGRAVE MACMILLAN is the global academic imprint of the Palgrave Macmillan division of St. Martin's Press, LLC and of Palgrave Macmillan Ltd. Macmillan® is a registered trademark in the United States, United Kingdom and other countries. Palgrave is a registered trademark in the European Union and other countries.

ISBN 0–333–80229–2 paperback

This book is printed on paper suitable for recycling and made from fully managed and sustained forest sources.

A catalogue record for this book is available from the British Library.

10   9   8   7   6   5   4   3   2   1
11   10   09   08   07   06   05   04   03   02

Printed and bound in Great Britain by J. W. Arrowsmith Ltd., Bristol

Contents

List of tables

List of contributors

The production of this book has involved its own division of labour. Davina Allen wrote Chapters 2, 7 and 8 and co-authored Chapter 4 with Morag Prowse. David Hughes wrote Chapter 1 and co-authored Chapter 3 with Sherrill Snelgrove and Chapter 6 with Sue Jordan. Davina Allen and David Hughes wrote Chapter 5.

Series editors' preface

It is widely accepted that because sociology can provide nurses with valuable and pertinent insights, it should be a constituent part of nursing's knowledge base. To take but a few substantive examples, sociology can help nurses understand the causes and distribution of ill health, the experience of health, illness and disability, the dynamics of health care encounters and the possibilities and limitations of professional care. Equally important, sociology's emphasis on critical reflection can encourage nurses to be more questioning and self-aware, thus helping them to provide flexible, non discriminatory, client-centred care in varied situations. Unfortunately, while the aspiration of integrating sociology into nursing knowledge is easy enough to state in theory, in practice the relationship has not been as productive as some might have anticipated. Notwithstanding a number of works which have successfully applied sociological tools to nursing problems, there remains a gulf between the two disciplines which has led some to question the utility of the relationship.

On the one hand, sociologists, while taking an interest in nursing's occupational position, have not paid great attention to the actual work that nurses do. This is partially due to the limitations of sociological surveillance. Nurses work in confidential, private and intimate settings with their clients. Sociologists' access to such settings is necessarily restricted. Moreover, nurses find it difficult to talk about their work, except to other nurses. As a result, core issues pertaining to nursing have been less than thoroughly treated in the sociological literature. There is thus a disjunction between what nurses require from sociology and what sociologists can provide.

On the other hand, nurses are on equally uncertain ground when they attempt to use sociology themselves. Often, nurses are reliant on carefully simplified introductory texts which, because of their broad remit, are often unable to provide in-depth understanding of sociological insights. Nor is it simply a matter of knowledge; there are tensions between the outlooks of nursing and sociology. Because nursing work involves individual interactions, it is not surprising that when nurses turn to sociology, they often turn to those elements which concentrate on micro-social interaction. While this is useful, in so far as it goes, it does not provide nurses with knowledge of the restraints and enablements imposed upon individual actions by social structures.

The aim of the *Sociology and Nursing Practice* series is to bridge these gaps between the disciplines. The authors of the series are nurses or teachers of nurses and therefore have an intimate understanding of nursing work and an appreciation of the importance of individualised nursing care. At the same time they are committed to a sociological outlook that asserts the salience of wider social forces to the work of nurses. The texts apply sociological theories and concepts to practical aspects of nursing. They explore nursing care as part of the social world, showing how different approaches to understanding the relationship between the individual and society have implications for nursing practice. By concentrating on specific concepts and drawing on research informed by social theory and methods, each book is able to provide the reader with a deeper understanding of the social construction of nurses' work. We hope the series will encourage nurses to analyse critically their practice and profession and to develop their own contribution to health and social care.

Margaret Miers, Sam Porter and Geoff Wilkinson

Acknowledgements

The research studies on which this book is based would not have been possible without the participation of a range of healthcare professionals, patients and carers. We thank them for so generously giving of their time in order that we might understand better their social worlds.

Chapter 2 is based on research funded by a Department of Health Nursing and Therapists Research Training Studentship. It reflects the author's opinion and does not represent the view of the Department of Health. The research was supervised by Professor Robert Dingwall (School of Sociology and Social Policy) and Professor Veronica James (School of Nursing), University of Nottingham.

The second of the research studies reported in Chapter 3 was funded by the Wales Office of Research and Development in Health and Social Care. Thanks are due to Jackie Lucas and Mike McIvor who provided assistance with the interviews utilised in this chapter. The views contained herein are those of the authors.

The doctoral research on which Chapter 4 is based was supervised by Professor Patricia Lyne School of Nursing and Midwifery Studies, University of Wales College of Medicine.

We are grateful to Margaret Miers and Geoff Wilkinson for their helpful comments on draft versions of the text and to Richie Hart, who so uncomplainingly provided IT emergency services.

This book contains material which has appeared in a different form elsewhere. Chapter 8: Allen D (2000) Negotiating the role of *expert carers* on an adult hospital ward. *Sociology and Health and Illness* 22(2): 149–71, is included by permission of Blackwell Publishers. Helpful comments on earlier drafts of the paper that formed the basis of this chapter were made by Patricia Lyne, Philip Burnard, Pat Jones, Carl May, the editors of *Sociology of Health and Illness* and two anonymous reviewers.

Davina Allen and David Hughes

Notes on contributors

Davina Allen is a Senior Lecturer and Deputy Director of the Nursing, Health and Social Care Research Centre, School of Nursing and Midwifery Studies, University of Wales College of Medicine. She has research interests in the social organisation of health and social care work, interface management and the sociology of organisations. She is the author of *The Changing Shape of Nursing Practice* (Routledge).

David Hughes is a Professor in the School of Health Science at University of Wales, Swansea. His research interests are in the fields of the healthcare division of labour, resource allocation, and comparative health care systems.

Sue Jordan holds a lecturership in the School of Health Science, University of Wales, Swansea. She is the author of a recent text on *Pharmacology for Midwives* (Palgrave), and is carrying out research in the two areas of chronic illness and educational evaluation.

Sherrill Snelgrove is a lecturer in the School of Health Science, University of Wales, Swansea. Her current research is on inter-professional relations and health psychology.

Morag Prowse is Head of Department, Clinical Studies in Adult Nursing, Institute of Health Studies, University of Plymouth. Her teaching interests include clinical practice, biosciences, inter-professional education, problem based learning, management, policy and evidence based health care.

1 Nursing and the division of labour: sociological perspectives

David Hughes

Introduction

The division of labour is a classic sociological concept with considerable contemporary relevance for nursing and other healthcare professions. In this book we hope to show that it provides a framework for linking a variety of recent developments – such as changes in occupational roles, skill-mix, educational preparation and professional regulation – with more global issues of social solidarity, legitimacy, power and social conflict. Nurses working in Western healthcare systems at the start of the twenty-first century find themselves in a period of rapid and sometimes turbulent organisational change. Often, it is not clear whether this represents an opportunity for professional advancement or a threat to existent professional norms and working conditions. Thus, in the UK the recent proliferation of nurse practitioner and expanded nursing roles has been portrayed both as a route to increased autonomy and status, and an attempt to cast nurses in the role of 'mini-doctors', who will be under medical control and lose touch with the core ideals of nursing work. Which view is correct? Although social science writings do not provide the one right answer to these questions, they offer conceptual frameworks that can sharpen debates and set recent changes in historical and comparative contexts. In this case they might alert us to the fact that occupations are not static entities, that work boundaries do change, that these changes are generally associated with negotiation or conflict with cognate occupations, and that the outcome in terms of the working relationships and relative standings of the occupations involved will depend on a range of structural, political and contingent factors.

This book sets out to explore some of the issues surrounding the healthcare division of labour by describing a series of research projects undertaken by the authors, in some cases in collaboration with colleagues. The unifying thread that runs through these investigations is that, in many settings throughout the contemporary UK National Health Service (NHS), occupational identities and practices are being reappraised in the light of wider organisational and technological change. Sometimes this involves a redrawing of occupational boundaries and a re-allocation, or expansion, of work that has consequences for the way nurses and others in associated occupations define their respective roles. Elsewhere, however, traditional inter-professional relationships persist even as other facets of the work change. This means that there is considerable empirical variation in the nature of inter-professional relationships in different work settings and clinical areas, some of which are documented in this volume. It would be an exaggeration to present these preliminary studies as a systematic programme of research, but most have origins in our longstanding interest in inter-professional relations and have been influenced by our common reading of the sociological literature on the division of labour.

There is of course a very large literature in this field and, in setting out the background for the particular research-based studies included in this book, we have been forced to be selective. There is, for example, no space here to review the full range of scholarship on managerialism and professionalism that has undoubted relevance to the contemporary division of labour, though one of us has produced a recent review of this material elsewhere (Allen 2001a: 1–21). Rather than aiming for complete coverage, we will discuss some of the key images or metaphors that have shaped social science thinking about these issues. To the extent that nurses and other healthcare workers are familiar with this literature we suspect that most see the division of labour through the twin prisms of professional struggle and gender relations, the frameworks that we will consider first. These approaches gained influence in the 1970s and 1980s at a time when many social scientists were preoccupied with conflict perspectives and the extension of patriarchy into the occupational domain. Most readers will know less about a second tradition that considers the division of labour in terms of the interdependence of occupations in a wider social system. We examine an early version of this approach represented by Emile Durkheim's notion of the 'social body', before considering the image of the division of labour as an aspect of a social ecological system. Towards the end of the chapter we introduce our case studies, and describe the methodological approach adopted.

Professional struggle

For many beginning students of the division of labour the primary metaphor is professional struggle, and the key concept is 'professional dominance'. Professional dominance is a theory about doctors and their control over healthcare work. It was developed by Freidson (1970a,b) from his work on the sociology of professions, and stemmed from his analysis of doctors' control of other categories of healthcare workers, such as nurses, midwives radiographers and pharmacists. Freidson sees all these occupations as paramedical professions – professions 'organised around the work of healing which are ultimately controlled by physicians'. They stand in an ambiguous relationship with medicine. On the one hand, they pose a threat because they have the potential to become healing consultancies that compete with doctors' practices. Yet, on the other hand, the services of such occupations are useful to medical professionals. They have traditionally provided a channel for delegating low status or routine work downwards, and take responsibility for specialist care services. Even though they constitute a potential threat to professional monopoly, it is not in the interest of the medical profession for them to disappear. Instead, the profession attempts to control their activities to protect its own position.

Freidson lists four aspects of this control. First, the technical knowledge learned and used by paramedical workers tends to be discovered, enlarged upon and approved by doctors. Second, the activities performed by paramedical workers ordinarily assist rather than replace the focal tasks of diagnosis and treatment. Third, paramedical workers are usually subordinate to doctors in the health division of labour. Finally, the prestige assigned by the general public to the paramedical workers is typically less than that given to the doctor. Freidson states that:

> In the medical organisation the medical profession is dominant. This means that all the work done by other occupations and related to the service of the patient is subject to the order of the physician. The profession alone is held competent to diagnose illness, treat or direct the treatment of illness, and evaluate the service. Without medical authorization little can be done for the patient by paraprofessional workers. (Freidson 1970b: 141)

Freidson argues that professional dominance has a number of overlapping dimensions. It is not simply a matter of subordination to an office holder who occupies a higher position in an organisational hierarchy, but also to authority based on the putatively superior knowledge of the professional expert.

Larkin (1983) accepts Freidson's view of the hierarchy of health occupations but places more emphasis on negotiated power. He argues that Freidson describes dominance rather than analysing control. The latter is usually not about open coercion but the ability to manage relations with other occupations in ways that preserve the medical profession's preeminent position. Larkin concedes that paramedical professions have been unsuccessful in achieving dominance over other groups, but argues that they have carved out secure occupational niches that they are well able to defend. While not disputing their place in the existing hierarchy, paramedical workers have scope to negotiate role boundaries with the medical profession so as to advance their relative position. Larkin suggests that, if the professional dominance thesis is taken to mean that the medical profession always gets its way, the significance of 'paramedical stratagems' will be seriously underestimated.

Freidson's reference to the 'putatively superior knowledge' of professional experts points to an important issue. Sometimes a paraprofessional worker is more knowledgeable about some aspect of the work than the doctor. Such a situation can lead to tensions because it creates an anomaly within the system of dominance. Even at the time of Freidson's early studies of professional power, other researchers reported a gap between formal organisational structures and informal practices which meant that subordinate occupations possessed considerable discretion to exert influence in certain areas of patient care (Mechanic 1961; Scheff 1961; Rushing 1965). Stein (1967) described how junior doctors and experienced nurses acted out a 'doctor/nurse game', whereby the nurse provided subtle cues to guide the neophyte physician, while preserving the fiction that care was determined by the doctor's instructions. As time passed there were suggestions that the nature of the 'game' might be changing under the influence of wider changes in Western healthcare systems, care technologies and social values (Stein *et al.* 1990). More recent studies have documented a continuum of practice ranging from the traditional superordinate/subordinate relationship, through disguised influence, to more overt challenges by nurses to doctors' authority (Hughes 1988; Porter 1991, 1995; Mackay 1993; Walby and Greenwell *et al.* 1994; Wicks 1998; Snelgrove and Hughes 2000). This research raises the question of how the changes that are occurring at the boundaries between medicine and nursing are experienced by participants. Svensson (1996) argues that the day-to-day division of labour between hospital doctors and nurses can be seen as a 'negotiated order' in which the lines of demarcation may be subject to ongoing changes. However, Allen's (1997) research in a provincial general hospital suggested that rather little negotiation regarding boundaries occurred at the face-to-face level of routine ward work, and that the boundary changes that were occurring related more clearly to understandings reached in higher level professional or management meetings. Given the internal diversity of modern healthcare systems and the heterogeneity of the settings involved, there are obvious dangers in generalising from single case studies, and this is clearly an area where more research is needed.

Larkin's (1983) study remains important as one of the few accounts we have of higher-level, formal negotiations affecting professional boundaries. However, he concentrates mainly on occupations such as ophthalmic opticians, radiographers and physiotherapists, which have been relatively successful in defending their place in the division of labour and a monopoly over special skills. He does not analyse the position of nurses, who for the most part have still not achieved independent practitioner status. Until recently, little formal negotiation, of the kind described by Larkin, appears to have occurred between nursing and the medical profession. However, this appears to be changing in the light of workforce constraints and workload pressures now affecting the NHS, which have led Governments to press the medical profession to concede more territory to nursing.

In the early 1990s concerns about the excessive hours worked by junior hospital doctors and the perceived need for a 'nursing contribution' to the problem, resulted in increased political support for expanded nursing roles. Since then the numbers of nurses receiving advanced training as clinical nurse specialists or nurse practitioners has risen sharply. There have also been moves to change the legal framework for drug prescribing. Following consultation on the second Crown Report (Department of Health 1999, 2000b, 2001; Medicines Control Agency 2001), nurses' involvement in the prescription of patients' medications seems likely to expand. With the support of the Royal College of Nursing (RCN), the UK Department of Health is committed to extending prescribing rights for some 200 prescription only medicines, and all pharmacy only and general sale items, to nurses completing a specified education programme. With most of these initiatives, consultation between the government and the key professions at the national level is followed by detailed negotiations at the local level. Thus, locally-agreed patient group directions have superseded 'standing orders' for group protocol prescribing, for example for analgesia in labour. These are negotiated amongst clinicians to reflect local conditions. On the whole, medical opposition to these developments has been muted, but the new arrangements often follow a pattern whereby medicine unburdens itself of 'tasks', while retaining overall clinical control, as, for example, with the proposed system (Crown II) of dependent and independent prescribers.[1]

Alongside the move into traditional medical territory, an alternative professionalising impulse has emerged in nursing. Rather than seeking professional status by taking on doctor-devolved work, many nurse leaders have pursued a policy of 'different but equal'. Thus, care activities that were initially devolved to health care assistants (HCA) as part of the re-allocation of tasks are now being redefined as high status work central to nursing's jurisdiction. For some, this has become part of a wider project to develop a distinct epistemology, different from that of medicine, and incorporating new conceptions of nursing knowledge, nursing classification and nursing diagnosis. This stance has its corollary in feminist critiques of professions and the division of labour.

The division of labour as patriarchy

Feminist analysis provides a useful corrective to the tendency to see the professionalisation process in terms of the natural histories of the classic male professions. Witz (1992) has suggested that sociology has been too quick to interpret the successful professional projects of certain class-based male occupations at a particular point in history as the paradigmatic model of profession. She argues that British nursing leaders have adopted a strategy of 'dual-closure', seeking on the one hand to resist domination from the medical profession and extend nursing territory, and on the other hand to regulate entry and defend the jurisdiction of the emergent nursing profession. While the campaign that culminated in the Nursing Registration Act of 1919 failed to bring nurses autonomous professional status, Witz argues that nursing's professionalising project re-emerged in the 1980s with the *Project 2000* reforms (UKCC 1987). This now incorporated a new emphasis on the content of nursing work, which Witz sees as a bid to establish practitioner autonomy over routine work that may well be successful.

The drive for professional status, and the competing visions of nursing that have emerged, create difficult dilemmas for feminist scholars. Some have argued that the best strategy for occupational advancement is to emphasise nursing's feminine qualities, based on the unique caring and nurturing capacities of women (Oakley 1984; Davies 1995). But others have cautioned that this approach risks trapping men and women in stereotyped gender roles (Savage 1987), and does nothing to counter the devaluation of basic caring skills (MacPherson

1991). Historically, gender has been both a resource and a liability for nursing (Gamarnikow 1991); it justifies the occupation's claims to jurisdiction over caring work but consigns it to a subordinate position *vis-à-vis* medicine. This legacy will not be easy to shake off.

Feminist writers share some common ground with conflict theorists like Freidson (such as the concern with power relations), but criticise 'malestream' sociology for paying insufficient attention to the gendered nature of healthcare work. Thus, it can be argued that although Freidson made much of medical control of the 'focal tasks' of diagnosis and treatment, much routine healthcare work is excluded from his analysis. In fact, contrary to Freidson's claims about the all-encompassing scope of medical supervision, there is little direct interference in routine ward management or 'hands-on' care activities. The dynamics of control of this work, without the need for professional oversight, is an important topic in its own right, but these activities remain invisible because of their low status as viewed through the gendered medical lens.

Davies (1995) has argued that healthcare organisations are shaped by cultural codes of masculinity and femininity that are deeply embedded in their design and functioning. Conceived in this way, organisations are not collections of neutral job positions occupied by people with gendered identities. Rather, they must be seen as social constructions that build organisational hierarchies, tasks and skills around gender difference, and rely on masculine values to make sense of organisational arrangements. Davies argues that even at the taken-for-granted level of the conceptualisation of jobs in bureaucratic organisations there are built-in requirements, such as the assumption of unencumbered work commitment, which give men an advantage over women. Thus, many successful male professionals or managers who conform to these occupational norms do so partly because their female partners are prepared to accept a supporting role, mirroring the traditional patriarchal family organisation.

According to Davies, women's supporting role is not confined to the domestic arena, but has been built into the gendered organisation of institutions such as the health service. The NHS contains many posts that function to support the (predominantly male) senior professionals and managers.

There are large numbers of clerks, HCAs, and other support workers who 'direct traffic' by moving patients and relatives through the system. Although having aspirations to professional status, nurses continue to be involved in this 'adjunct work', which is seen as supplementary to the expert work of the core professionals.

[T]he work process can often only be accomplished in the requisite detached and impersonal manner by dint of a great deal of preparatory and serving work which is carried out only by women. Women are the first points of contact with the client. Often it is women who are there, both before and after, attending to the 'detail' which processes and shaped the client so that the professional interaction can take place. Women also attend not only to the informational, but the physical and emotional needs of the bureaucrat, the professional and the client, sustaining a sense of order, and handling tension. This work is rarely acknowledged or well conceptualised: from the point of view of the gendered professional ideal it is regarded as trivial or as 'support'. (Davies 1995: 61)

These female workers develop a range of co-ordination skills, which bring order to a system otherwise made up of specialists who are responsible for specific tasks in specific locations on the 'healthcare assembly line'. However, this contribution remains unrecognised and poorly rewarded. Indeed feminist critics have argued that skills are not an objective economic fact, but an 'ideological category' influenced by the relative power of gendered occupational groups (Phillips and Taylor 1980; Davies and Rosser 1986). Since many of the tasks undertaken by female employees are defined as 'natural' work for women – an extension of the normal domestic role – they are not seen as skilled work (Needleman and Nelson 1988).

Feminist writers also note that 'malestream' sociologists have been slow to analyse the relationship between formal healthcare and informal domestic care (Stacey 1988). Although a great deal of health work straddles this boundary, it remained as invisible as the routine hospital work mentioned above. Early work on informal care tends to focus on the unpaid work of female carers (Ungerson 1983; Graham 1985). It was argued that the shift of healthcare resources into community and primary care worked to increase the burden falling on women in the home (Gregor 1997). In recent years it has become clear that almost as many men as women take on responsibilities as informal carers (Rose and Bruce 1995; Arber and Gilbert 1989), and there is an increasing recognition that the professional/lay interface is shaped by a range of cultural and social factors.

There are many facets of feminist analysis that we have no space to discuss here, and indeed this is the topic of a companion volume in this series (Miers 2000). The significance of gender for labour market processes has been documented by a number of researchers (Carpenter 1993; Crompton and Sanderson 1990; Evans 1997; Gamarnikow 1978, 1991; Walby 1989; Witz 1986, 1988, 1992). While we believe that feminist researchers have sometimes been guilty of taking a uni-focal approach and overstating their position, their work contributes many valuable insights. In particular they remind us of the gendered nature of healthcare organisations and the sociological neglect of much routine healthcare work. Feminist research suggests that a proper analysis of the healthcare division of labour needs to incorporate the full range of occupations, tasks and skills that are implicated in the care process, including the informal caring that intersects with paid health work.

Durkheim and the social body

Recent social conflict approaches bear a family resemblance to earlier social theory that linked the growth of the division of labour to the interests of particular social groups. In the writings of Marx and Weber increasing specialisation was seen as a corollary of capitalism and the growth of markets. The rapidly changing division of labour disrupted traditional communities and led to the increasing isolation and alienation of individual workers. But this view was quickly challenged by other commentators of the time, including the nineteenth-century French sociologist Emile Durkheim. While many of his contemporaries were preoccupied with occupational specialisation as a manifestation of mechanisation and the concentration of capital, and a source of social dislocation and conflict, Durkheim was interested in the question of how differentiation might co-exist with social solidarity. His classic study, *The Division of Labour in Society*, was concerned with the persistence of integrative norms and co-operative behaviour, even where specialised occupational roles had developed. Durkheim tried to understand the division of labour in terms of the biological metaphor of the organism. The 'social body' resembles organisms in which specialised sub-systems perform different functions:

[T]he law of the division of labour applies to organisms as to societies: it can even be said that the more specialised the functions of the organism, the greater its development. [...] It is no longer considered only a social institution that has its source in the intelligence and will of men, but is a phenomenon of general biology whose conditions must be sought in the essential properties of organised matter. (Durkheim 1933: 41) (First French edition, 1893)

Durkheim argued that the move to modern forms of economic organisation did not eradicate social ties, but itself created new sources of social solidarity to replace those that were being swept away. In traditional societies members were united by similarity, based on factors such as kinship and social rank. The form of social solidarity that existed was 'mechanical', in the sense that moral obligations are experienced as 'natural' and associated with ascribed status in a taken-for-granted way. However, under modern conditions of specialisation a new form of organic solidarity based on differences emerges. Durkheim took issue with economic liberals who saw the individual pursuit of self-interest within markets as the basis of social order. Economic calculations of interest, as reflected in contractual exchange and the underpinning legal framework, did not seem to him to provide a stable basis for co-operative behaviour over time. For Durkheim, the operation of contracts depended on an unwritten substratum of norms and mutual obligations – the so-called non-contractual basis of contract. This was a precondition for the mutual trust on which business relationships depended, and which would ensure that contracts were honoured. Thus, modern capitalist societies depended on a moral order, though not one based on the ascriptive ties that operated prior to the agrarian and industrial revolutions. It was the division of labour that, according to Durkheim, created the web of mutual obligation that enabled a market system to function. The increasing differentiation of human endeavours contributes to social cohesion because accentuated difference increases interdependence and the need for co-operation. Individuals performing strikingly different tasks must find a structure in which they depend for some things on others if their needs are to be met. Durkheim sought to explain societal change in terms of social rather than individual factors, and this may have led him to construct an image of the normative and moral order that has been widely criticised by modern social theorists (see, e.g. Fletcher 1971). At times, Durkheim comes close to regarding society as a kind of 'super-organic entity' with a life and consciousness of its own. Rather than conceding a role for individual consciousness and purpose, Durkheim uses concepts such as 'collective representations', 'collective sentiments', and elements of 'collective conscience' to relate the moral order to the social body as a whole. The idea of a long-term trend towards greater specialisation is central to Durkheim's notion of the 'progress of the division of labour'. He posited that more developed societies would be characterised by increased specialisation: 'If one takes away the various forms the division of labour assumes according to conditions of time and place, there remains the fact that it advances regularly in history' (Durkheim 1933: 233). Among other things, increased specialisation is caused by a rise in 'moral' and 'material' density. Greater numbers of people are brought into close proximity, they establish social relations, and this interaction increases the web of mutual interdependence. Durkheim also recognised the possibility that occupational competition could accelerate this process. Drawing on Darwinian theory, he argued that in circumstances where similar enterprises struggled for survival in competition with each other, some might have no alternative but to disappear or transform, and such transformations often led to new specialisms. In Durkheim's view this rarely involved a 'fight to the finish', but rather a re-allocation of functions as successful enterprises expanded their operations to take in new tasks and weaker ones retrenched to concentrate on only a part of the work they previously undertook.

Although now more than a century old, Durkheim's writings still provide many important insights into contemporary policy processes. His ideas on the integrative ties of the underlying

moral order remind us that, for most of the time in most arenas of society, the division of labour rests on a fair measure of
co-operation and mutual interdependence. The related notion
of the 'non-contractual' basis of contract has become especially topical as a powerful counterpoint to the economic lib-
eralism that has helped shape recent health reforms in many
countries. Several accounts of the recent NHS reforms, which
are concerned with the tension between professional norms
and the 1990s discourse of markets and competition, rely on
essentially Durkheimian arguments (e.g. Ferlie 1994; Flynn *et al.*
1996; Hughes 1996).

However, the major weakness of Durkheim's underlying
organic metaphor is that it leads us to think about societies in
much the same way that we think about biological entities.
Later generations of social scientists have questioned the
applicability of Darwinist theory to the social domain, and
Durkheim's notion of 'collective conscience' has also lost
credibility. The idea of the social body as a biological system
leads to a preoccupation with the functions of the parts, and
limits the scope for theorising about how systems can change
and develop. Later theorists sought to develop an approach
that recognised the importance of studying the interrelations
between social groups and institutions in a wider field of
action, but jettisoned the image of the social body and its
underlying functionalist assumptions.

Social ecological theory

Early social ecological writings represented a shift of emphasis
rather than a sharp break with the Durkheimian approach.
The language of 'function' and even of 'organ' was still sometimes present, but the focus shifted from the single organism
(the 'social body') to a multiplicity of social organs and their
ecology. The Chicago sociologist, Everett Hughes wrote that:

> The division of labour represents a series of exchanges between com-
> munities whereby these communities become involved as functioning
> parts of a larger community. This larger community, however, has
> no common conscience, or only a very tenuous, abstract one. As
> the division of labour proceeds, the life of each social organ is more

conditioned by the others; the forces which hold it in place come to include neighbours as well as the soil beneath one's feet. It is this pattern of social organs, treated spatially, with which human ecology concerns itself. (Hughes 1984: 328)

Hughes refers approvingly to Durkheim's work, but in practice puts more emphasis on the dynamics of ecological systems than on the functions of parts. Much of Hughes's writing is cast in the language of 'institutions', by which he refers to recurrent patterns of social action that take on the character of social structures, such as the various occupations that make up the division of labour. He argues that the study of institutions concerns the contingencies 'that arise out of the inevitable relations of social phenomena with other social phenomena and with phenomena that are not social at all' (1984: 6). Thus, among other things, the survival of institutions is bound up with succession in space, the movements of people and the changing nature of collective wants. Over time, institutions compete for space, clientele and legitimacy in ways that depend critically on their local environments and their interactions with other institutions. It was these 'spatial contingencies' (1984: 13) in particular that provided a focus for Hughes's work and the ecological approach.

Hughes made an analytic distinction between the role and task components of occupations. The 'technical division of labour' refers to the allocation of tasks ('what I do'), while the moral division of labour refers to the allocation of roles ('who I am'). For Hughes, an occupation consists of a bundle of tasks, which are shaped by both technical and role factors. Sometimes the tasks are strongly identified with a given occupational role and its claim to certain skills, but in other cases tasks have been bundled together for reasons of history or convenience. Occupational members may value certain task components, while considering others to be 'dirty' work. The bundles of tasks are not fixed, but may change as a result of other shifts in the system of work.

Hughes emphasised that both tasks and roles change in light of contingent factors, which may set up tensions between the technical and moral divisions of labour:

[I]n the medical world there are two contrary trends operating simultaneously. As medical technology develops and changes, particular tasks are constantly downgraded; that is, they are delegated by the physician to the nurse. The nurse in turn passes them to the maid. But occupations and people are being upgraded within certain limits. The nurse moves up nearer the doctor in techniques and devotes more of her time to supervision of other workers. [...] And the question arises of the effect of changes in technical division upon the roles involved. (Hughes 1984: 307–8)

In Hughes's view, the process by which occupations took on valued new tasks, while delegating unwanted tasks to others was an important prerequisite for occupational mobility. Hughes sees nursing as an occupation that is seeking to gain recognition as a profession. He correctly predicts other developments such as the move of nursing into university education, and the emergence of nursing research and higher degrees, which he links to this professionalising project (see Hughes 1958, Chapter 10). What Hughes failed to anticipate, however, was that professionalisation projects could also be based on a feminist-inspired challenge to the medical skills hierarchy of the kind outlined earlier.

A theme to which Hughes constantly returned was that the work of a particular occupation could only be understood as part of a wider social system. For Hughes, the social system was not just the players at the centre of the stage (say, the doctor and patient) but the wider 'institutional matrix' within which the work takes place:

Every one or nearly every one of the many important services given by professionals in our times is given in a complex institutional setting. The professional must work with a host of non-professionals (and the professionals are normally short-sighted enough to use that pejorative term *ad naseum*). These other workers bring into the institutional complex their own conceptions of what the problem is, their own conceptions of their rights and privileges, and their careers and life-fate. (Hughes 1984: 310)

Thus, the study of the division of labour involved an examination of the system of work from the perspectives of many kinds of workers, high and low, and at the periphery as well as the centre of events.

The importance of spatial metaphors in social ecological theory is illustrated by the work of Dingwall and associates (Dingwall 1983; Dingwall and Lewis 1983; Dingwall *et al.* 1988). Dingwall draws a parallel between Chicago studies of work and occupations and contemporaneous studies of urban life.

> The world of work was treated as an analogue to the city of Chicago urban ecology. A given terrain of demands for goods and services was divided into blocks of tasks, which might be developed, redeveloped or extinguished. These blocks had successive occupiers, competing for access and struggling to improve their status by new acquisitions or the relinquishment of less attractive properties. (Dingwall 1983)

He argues that the study of the division of labour needs to start by considering the work that must be done. Over time, it is the work – the core activities that society needs to get done – that is the most stable variable. Taking this as the starting point one can go on to ask how various occupations form, how they divide the work and how this division of labour changes over time. This can be compared to the development of a city. One can think of the totality of work needing to be done as the land on which the city is built. The different occupations can be seen as buildings erected on the land. The point is that cities are not static. As redevelopment occurs, buildings may be enlarged. Sometimes buildings are demolished and new ones built. The development of new areas of work can be compared to the outward spread of the city, or the filling in of pockets of land that had previously remained undeveloped. As the nature of the work changes, the boundaries of occupations also shift. They may fuse or divide, and sometimes tasks previously carried out by one occupation may be passed onto another (see also Dingwall *et al.* 1988).

The most influential recent exposition of social ecological theory comes in Abbott's (1988) *The System of Professions: An Essay on the Division of Expert Labour*. According to Abbott, earlier theories of professionalisation, preoccupied as they were with the form of professions (trait theory) and their structural position in society (functionalist and conflict theories), paid insufficient attention to the content of professional work. Yet, it is the content rather than the form of professional work that is changing, Abbott claims. He proposes that the proper unit of analysis should be the professional task area, which he calls 'jurisdiction'. In his view it is the interaction between occupations as they struggle for control over this task area that is critical: he argues that the evolution of professions results from their interrelations and that the proper subject for study is therefore the wider system of professions.

Abbott argues that each profession is bound to a set of tasks by jurisdictional ties, and the development of professions is centrally implicated with the creation of these ties. Jurisdiction has both cultural and structural aspects. The cultural dimension is concerned with how tasks are constructed as professional problems. Professions do not seek to control the work by controlling technique, but by developing a body of abstract knowledge which incorporates the profession's special expertise and norms. Jurisdiction also has a social structure. Jurisdictional claims arise in different ways in public, legal and workplace arenas. The public arena is important in establishing the profession's symbolic claims over an area of work, and the legal arena guarantees the profession's formal control and defines the precise boundaries of its jurisdiction. However, it is in the work setting that the details of jurisdiction are worked out in face-to-face social interactions. This is the level where formalised job descriptions are translated into actual working relationships, on the basis of negotiation and custom.

Abbott argues that jurisdictional boundaries are in constant dispute, both in local practice and national inter-professional politics. Most professions desire full jurisdiction. However, because professions are part of a system, there are not enough full jurisdictions to go around and most must seek a partial settlement. Such settlements can take many forms. There may be a division of labour according to tasks or clientele, or a form of delegation where one profession advises but does not control another, or the subordination of one profession to another. Abbott suggests that the position of nursing in relation to medicine takes this latter form. He suggests that this form of subordination often involves fuzzy occupational boundaries that would be a threat if public and legal jurisdictions were not already established.

Abbott's thesis has other detailed elements that we have no space to treat here, and it clearly represents a plausible statement of aspects of the situation of modern nursing. The main limitations in terms of the development of social ecological theory are its restriction to the 'professions'. Thus, Abbott does not pay enough attention to Hughes's injunction to include the occupations which make up the wider institutional matrix within which the professions operate. Nor does he pay any attention to the unpaid work that supports the formal healthcare system. This is important for nursing work, where the boundaries between paid and unpaid caring are frequently blurred and subject to change over time. As one of us has argued elsewhere (Allen 2001a), it might be said that Abbott's work is both systematising and not systematising enough. If the analytic focus is to be restricted to professions then the limits of the system need to be more clearly specified. But given the notorious difficulty of defining 'profession' this may prove to be a problematic task, and we need to move beyond the system of professions to consider the system of work as a whole.

Studying the division of labour as social interaction

Although the four approaches discussed may sometimes appear to stand in tension, we believe that each contains valuable insights that are capable of synthesis (Allen 2001a). Certainly they did not evolve in isolation. The school of Chicago sociology that gave rise to the social ecological approach was influenced by Durkheim, and – through its association with the sociological perspective of symbolic interactionism – in turn influenced the work of Freidson. The conflict perspective with which Freidson's work became linked influenced feminist perspectives, which also made use of qualitative methods that had been brought back into prominence by neo-Chicago interactionist researchers. Moreover, although not treated well in terms of tenured positions, women made an important contribution in shaping the research programme and reformist stance of Chicago sociology during its golden period (Deegan 1995). Each of the approaches points to the importance of studying nursing work in the context of a wider division of labour and its relations with other occupations and informal carers. This leads to a common focus on social interaction as the process in which actors negotiate the nature of their working roles and relationships.

Changes in existing work organisation depend partly on macro-level developments, such as the passage of legislation that confirms or overturns professional monopoly powers, but also on the ability of occupations to advance their jurisdictional claims in interaction with other occupations. Inter-professional relations are thus a critical arena in which the existing division of labour is sustained, and is changed over time as new levers of influence are brought to bear. This is a key theme of the case studies contained in this book, which illustrate the tensions, conflict and accommodation observable when occupations, or sub-groups within occupations, come together to negotiate working relationships. Our concern is not with historical or structural accounts of occupational change but the significance of micro-level interactions in sustaining or changing an existing division of labour 'from the bottom up'. While the authors acknowledge the influence of 'macro' factors, we believe that there is a space for detailed case studies of intra-professional and inter-professional relations, of a kind that are currently rarely done.

The case studies that follow deal with a range of settings, but admittedly do not capture the full spectrum of role changes currently affecting the NHS. Our focus reflects the completed work of two small research groups in our respective institutions, and we acknowledge that we say little about important developments occurring in areas such as primary and community care, mental health, midwifery and child health. We concentrate mainly on hospital care, and mainly on the nursing/medical boundary, the boundary between nurses and HCAs, and the professional/lay interface. While we believe that many of the findings are generalisable to other contexts of inter-professional work, we recognise that the proper investigation of the health division of labour requires a much larger programme of work that will take researchers into many other settings.

Although each of the chapters is intended to be a free-standing account of a particular research project, they have been arranged to cover a series of overlapping topics concerning the division of labour. We start with three case studies based on observations and/or qualitative interviews. Chapter 2 examines the crucial significance of time and space in shaping nursing work in a general hospital, paying special attention to its consequences for the division of labour between nurses, doctors and HCAs. Chapter 3 describes how both hospital doctors and nurses express a commitment to new patterns of team working, but turn out on closer inspection to be operating with very different ideas of what is involved and what this means for traditional occupational hierarchies. Chapter 4 takes us into the special locale of the post-anaesthesia care unit (PACU) to examine nurses' contrasting accounts of their relations with doctors in routine work interactions and emergency situations. These narratives suggest a real change in behaviour where nurses respond to emergencies by adopting a more assertive, directive approach to patient care, but they also shed light on the 'moral realities' surrounding the division of labour, in terms of the justifications or grounds that nurses invoke when they move into the doctors' territory.

In Chapter 5 we step back from the specifics of particular settings to present findings from a survey of junior doctors', nurses' and HCAs' views of expanded nursing role developments. While we found an unexpected strength of opposition to expanded roles in the nursing profession itself, we argue that this is not so much a reflection of nursing's 'conservatism' as part of the natural dynamics of an organisational change process in which stakeholders seek to clarify both intended and unintended consequences. Chapter 6 draws on a mixture of survey, interview and observational data to examine nurses' perceptions of the significance of advanced bioscience training for roles and professional relationships after the course was completed. While improved knowledge about medication monitoring sometimes led nurses into medical territory, this research suggests that it was the nursing hierarchy, rather than doctors, that did most to constrain significant role changes.

The final two chapters examine the professional/lay interface, again reporting findings from qualitative case studies. Chapter 7 explores how the division of labour between patients and their families on the one hand, and nurses on the other, are shaped by the 'contexts' of care (encompassing factors such as skill-mix and channels for information transmission). The reasons why a 'participatory caring context' was accomplished in one locale and not another are considered. Chapter 8, which draws on the same study, looks at expert carers and examines the tensions that influence their interactions with nursing staff. Both chapters make a case for a wider conceptualisation of the health division of labour, which includes both paid professionals and the informal care network.

We envisage that the text may be used in a number of ways. It is our aim that, taken as a whole, the book will provide an introduction to the theory and application of sociology to a key issue of concern for nurses. Nevertheless, because each of the chapters is freestanding, they can be read in isolation for their particular theoretical and substantive content. Moreover, although the papers draw on research in specific practice areas, they do have a broader value as stimulus material inviting comparison and contrast with other clinical settings. Finally, the chapters are intentionally data-rich; the empirical material can therefore be considered either in its own terms and/or in terms of its fit with the associated analysis.

2 Time and space on the hospital ward: shaping the scope of nursing practice

Davina Allen

Introduction

Time and space are among the core building blocks of any culture (Helman 1992). Since the beginning of the modern era, philosophers and scientists have insisted that time and space are essential concepts for comprehending the world and one's place within it (Gross 1982) and in the social sciences, the linkage of time and space has a long history (Friedland and Boden 1994; Glennie and Thrift 1996). There is, for example, a strong tradition of temporal–spatial analyses of work and the division of labour (Smith (1976) [1776]; Marx (1970) [1887]; Thompson 1967; Taylor 1975) which continues to flourish to this day (e.g. Malmberg 1995; Collinson and Collinson 1997). In medical sociology, moreover, the importance of temporal–spatial considerations in shaping the social organisation and experience of health and illness is increasingly being recognised (Davis 1956; Roth 1963; Frankenberg 1992; Zerubavel 1979a,b; Rosengren and DeVault 1963; Glaser and Strauss 1965, 1968; Strauss *et al.* 1985). In recent years, feminist scholars have underlined the relationship between time and gender (Davies 1989; Hochschild 1989; Adam 1995; Glucksmann 1995; Sullivan 1997) and have pointed to the consequences that this has for women's lives. My aim, in this chapter, is to illustrate how thinking in terms of space and time can shed some light on the work role of ward-based hospital nurses.

Orthodox analyses of nursing work have tended to emphasise the importance of wider social processes – such as professionalisation, gender (Witz 1986, 1988, 1992, 1994; Davies 1995; Wicks 1998) and economic factors (Dingwall *et al.*

1988) – in shaping the niche occupied by nursing within the healthcare system. Yet, while such macro-sociological considerations are clearly important for any understanding of nursing work, they are only part of the picture. To comprehend fully how the scope of nursing work is fashioned in *daily practice* we also need to look to key features of the work setting. In this chapter, I am going to examine how the temporal–spatial ordering of hospital settings shapes the contours of nursing work. Drawing on doctoral research into the ways in which nurses routinely managed occupational jurisdiction (Allen 1996, 1997, 1998, 2000a,b,c, 2001a,b; Allen and Lyne 1997), I focus on three key nursing boundaries: the intra-occupational division of labour and the nurse–support worker and nurse–doctor interfaces.

The study

The study was carried out on a medical ward and a surgical ward in a district general hospital in the middle of England. It had an annual budget of £60 million, almost 900 beds and 2800 staff, and provided general, acute, obstetric and elderly services to a local population of 254 000.

Ethnographic research methods were utilised: participant observation, informal conversations, semi-structured tape-recorded interviews with staff and documentary analysis of a range of organisational literature (patient information leaflets, memoranda, (anonymised) careplans and ward philosophies). Fieldwork was undertaken over a ten-month period. I am a nurse, but did not work in this capacity during the fieldwork, although I did participate in hospital life when it felt appropriate to do so. Overall, I was overt about my nursing background but emphasised and de-emphasised this aspect of my personal biography according to the demands of the fieldwork. My badge was inscribed with the title: 'research student'.

Three months were spent on each ward. I recorded my observations contemporaneously in a shorthand notebook. These were 'low inference' in style, that is, they were literal descriptions of field actors' behaviour and talk, rather than my interpretations or glossing of events. Certain activities were also tape-recorded: meetings, nursing handover and study days. The observational data were supplemented by semi-focused audio tape-recorded interviews. The interview sample comprised: ward nurses ($n = 29$), doctors ($n = 8$), auxiliaries ($n = 5$), health care assistants (HCAs) ($n = 3$) and clinical managers ($n = 11$). Data generation and analysis were undertaken concurrently, with analysis informing subsequent data collection. The study was guided by an interactionist theoretical framework (Strauss *et al.* 1963, 1964, 1985; Freidson 1976; Strauss 1978; Hughes 1984; Abbott 1988). The division of labour was conceptualised as in process, actively negotiated and re-negotiated within a given context and according to the purposes at hand.

An holistic approach to data analysis was adopted: data from different sources were compared in order to make judgements as to how each piece should be interpreted. Data extracts were cross-checked with the emergent overall analysis in order to evaluate their meaning. A broad coding frame was developed and subsequently modified as the analysis progressed. Folio VIEWS 3.1 was employed to facilitate data management and handling.

Time and space in the hospital context

Organisational challenges

> There are sacred, profane, metaphysical, biological and clock times, but we have little idea of how they all fit together or how each affects our lives [...] all of us [...] are tied together in an endless web of rhythms – rhythms that influence how [...] people relate to each other. (Hall 1983: 14)

As 'people-processing' organisations, hospitals bring together a multitude of interpenetrating physical, biological and cultural time frames (Adam 1995). For 365 days a year, they provide 24-hour care to a continuous throughput of biographically distinct individuals. All are at different stages in their illness (Strauss *et al.* 1985), recovery (Lawler 1991) or dying trajectory (Glaser and Strauss 1965, 1968) and each has unique bodily rhythms and temporal concerns (Roth 1963; Davis

1956; Strauss *et al.* 1985; Frankenberg 1992). Not only is this 'people-work' inherently unpredictable (Melia 1979; Strauss *et al.* 1985), managing multiple patient needs poses particular problems of organisation. One of the ways in which hospitals have dealt with this management challenge is by ordering patients in both time and space. As Glennie and Thrift (1996) argue, this kind of 'time-discipline' involves standardisation, regularity and co-ordination.

Standardisation

> Standardisation refers to 'the degree to which people's time–space paths are disciplined to be the same as one another's.' (Glennie and Thrift 1996: 285)

Inside the hospital, patients are categorised and allocated to pre-defined spaces, for the most part, according to their healthcare requirements. Various healthcare specialists coalesce within these different locales, bringing their skills to bear on the cases they encounter. The different 'workshops', to which patients may be allocated, each have a distinctive 'shape' (Strauss *et al.* 1985): they have developed their own divisions of labour, tempos and rhythms and definitions of 'routine' and 'emergency' according to their functions and the normal kinds of conditions which are usually handled there. Most recently, in the US and the UK standardisation has been taken to new extremes moving beyond the local to the national setting with the introduction of patient care pathways (Sulch and Kalra 2000) and the introduction of 'Clinical Governance' and 'National Service Frameworks' in the UK (Department of Health 1998a).

Regularity

> Regularity refers to 'the degree to which people's time–space paths involve repetitive routine'. (Glennie and Thrift 1996: 285)

A further way in which hospitals cope with the multiple temporal rhythms of their patient populations is through the introduction of a common timetable (Goffman 1961; Roth 1963; Bellaby 1992). Typical in other situations of 'batch-living', such as monasteries, this kind of set routine gives hospital work some predictability providing staff and patients (Roth 1963; Fairhurst 1977; Zerubavel 1979a) with a sort of 'repertoire' of what is expected, and what is likely to occur within certain temporal boundaries. While the total absence of predictability would be psychologically intolerable (Moore 1963), as a strategy for managing the collectivity, it is inevitable that these organisational routines will be out of synch with the personal routines and natural rhythms of individuals.

> [F]or the patients, the passage of time in hospital appears to continue inflexibly from routine with almost total disruption of the 'normal, natural' rhythms of bodily desires. (Frankenberg 1992: 4)

Co-ordination
Co-ordination refers to:

> the degree to which people's time–space paths are disciplined to smoothly connect to one another's. (Glennie and Thrift 1996: 285)

Over the course of a single in-patient episode patients move through different spaces within the hospital where they are attended to by a range of personnel. Emergency admissions, for example, will have their first contact with the hospital in the accident and emergency department. On arrival, they will be assessed (possibly by a triage nurse) and the urgency of their condition ranked against the overall workload of the department. They will then be allocated to 'resus' if necessary or, if not, a cubicle (if one is available). Here, they will wait until the doctor and other relevant health professionals have time to see them. Once the medical assessment has been made, then a number of alternatives are possible. It may be necessary for the patient to be transferred to the X-ray department for investigations or, in certain cases, immediate surgery may be indicated. Discharge home under the care of their general practitioner is another possibility, as is transfer to an admissions ward where further processing will take place before they are eventually admitted to a specialist ward. Over the course of their in-patient career, moreover, they may move both within and from 'their' ward to other hospital spaces according to their medical needs.

Ensuring the seamless and integrated provision of health-care services and a smooth passage between the 'variegated workshops' (Strauss *et al.* 1985) in this complex system presents particular challenges of co-ordination (see also Chapter 4, this volume). For example, although hospitals provide 24-hour care, some services are only available at certain times (Zerubavel 1979a). As a consequence, the respective temporal concerns of the various departments may be very different and, in some instances, their timetables can be asynchronous. In addition, there are also important issues of continuity. That is, how to ensure the communication of essential information as the patient passes through the various domains of the hospital and/or is attended to by different members of the healthcare team. It is here that the medical record plays a key role and, in recent years, there have been a number of developments directed at improving upon the extant system, such as multi-disciplinary case notes and patient-held records.

Power

Time and space are also integral to power relations within the hospital (Henley 1977; Tellis-Nayak and Tellis-Nayak 1984; Glucksmann 1998). Place is important in shaping our identities and in augmenting or undermining our sense of agency (Liaschenko 1994; Goffman 1961, Chapters 7 and 8 this volume).

> Removal of patients, whether male or female, to hospital or even to clinics, whether outpatient departments or consulting rooms of GPs, puts them in a space where the patients' uncertainty is reinforced by the certitudes of the physician's (and to a lesser extent other health workers') understanding of complicated routines. (Frankenberg 1992: 16–17)

Time and power are inextricably linked (Thompson 1967); when there is a need to co-ordinate multiple times then it becomes evident that not all times are equal (Adam 1995). We make fewer demands on the time of the powerful; the powerless are thought to have more time on their hands (Schwartz 1979; Tellis-Nayak and Tellis-Nayak 1984).

> In order to maintain social order and restore natural order, patients are removed from normal temporalities to a space where the time view of

others can be imposed upon them. [...] It iatrogenically produces a situation of enhanced power for the healers and reduced autonomy for
the patients. (Frankenberg 1992: 25)

Over the last decade, against a rising tide of consumer
consciousness, hospitals have been criticised for organising
their services for the convenience of the staff rather than the
patients (e.g. Department of Health & Social Security 1983).
In the UK, a range of initiatives, aimed *inter alia* at addressing the traditional asymmetries of power between healthcare
professionals and patients, have attended to issues of time and
space. For example, patients are now encouraged to get
dressed in the day rather than being stripped (metaphorically
and literally) of their identities on admission to hospital
(cf. Goffman 1961). With the liberalisation of visiting hours
the spaces of hospital wards are being increasingly opened up.
Patients' time is also being accorded greater value. Outpatients
are now given individual, rather than 'batch', appointments
and a whole range of easy-access consumer-style services –
such as NHS Direct and nurse-run drop-in centres – have been
introduced. In addition, care is increasingly being delivered in
the private spaces of patients' homes rather than the public
spaces of the hospital where the primacy of medical time is at
its zenith (Pritchard 1992). As yet, however, there is little
empirical evidence of the impact of community-based care on
the distribution of power relations in healthcare. Some have
seen these developments as having important implications for
shifting the ownership of time and space in favour of patients
(Glazer 1993; Allen 2000a). Others take a less sanguine view,
interpreting these trends as evidence of a further widening of
the medical gaze (Liaschenko 1994) and an extension of the
medicalisation of additional aspects of social life. Whatever the
effects of these changes in the temporal–spatial ordering of
healthcare on the power relations between health services
staff, one thing is clear: the shift towards community services
has also resulted in a redistribution of time from waged to
unwaged carers, with relatives and significant others now
expected to provide for dependant family members (e.g. Finch
1990; Ungerson 1990). As policy analysts have argued,
although the drive towards community care was motivated, in
part, by humanitarian concerns, the biggest impetus came

from the realisation that care *by* the community would be cheaper.

Time is money

What this last point illustrates is that in Western society 'time is money'. Control of time is an important part of industrial life (Starkey 1992) and a key task of management is to see that time is not wasted. As we enter the twenty-first century, modern healthcare systems appear to be caught between two contrary trends: the call for more individually focused services on the one hand, and the continued drive for increased efficiencies, on the other. In UK hospitals, patient throughput has escalated, raising acuity levels and the intensity and content of the work. At the same time, the division of labour in healthcare has been increasingly scrutinised in order to effect cost-savings and the health professions have been regularly criticised for maintaining inefficient demarcatory practices. As the largest occupational group in the health service, nursing has been particularly vulnerable to the 'new public management' (Hood 1991) gaze, frequently facing the charge that they could deploy their time to better effect (e.g. Health Services Management Unit 1996).

Managing monochronic and polychronic time

One way of understanding these strains in the temporal–spatial ordering of the hospital is in terms of the wider tensions in the time–space organisation of modern Western societies. Hall (1983) has identified two different ways in which complex societies organise time: monochronic and polychronic time. Monochronic time is linear: time is seen as stretching from past to future, subdivided into segments – years, hours and minutes – and social life is governed by 'tasks, schedules and procedures'. In societies dominated by monochronic time, a premium is placed on speed and doing more in less time. Hall argues that monochronic time scheduling makes it possible to compartmentalise and concentrate on only one thing at a time, but it also reduces the context.

Since scheduling by its very nature selects what will and will not be perceived and attended, and permits only a limited number of events within a given period, what gets scheduled constitutes a system for setting priorities for both people and functions. (Hall 1983: 53)

Thus, while monochronic time is an efficient form of social organisation and, as Hall argues, it is unlikely that without it industrial civilisation could have developed as it has (see also Thompson 1967), it is often blind to human needs. Polychronic time, by contrast, involves doing many things at once. Here the onus is placed on relations, and people and the completion of transactions rather than rigid schedules. Hall argues that:

Any human being who is naturally drawn to other human beings and who lives in a world dominated by human relationships will be either pushed or pulled toward the polychronic end of the spectrum. If you value people, you must hear them out and cannot cut them off simply because of a schedule. [...] [Monochronic time], on the other hand, is oriented to tasks, schedules, and procedures. As anyone who has had experience with our bureaucracies knows, schedules and procedures take on a life of their own without reference to either logic or human needs. (Hall 1983: 50)

These temporal systems are, according to Hall, logically and empirically distinct, 'like oil and water they do not mix' and yet in modern Western societies they are frequently embedded in each other (Davies 1989; Adam 1995; Glennie and Thrift 1996). Monochronic time dominates the public sphere, whereas polychronic time is the temporal form most commonly found in the private domain of the home. Given the gendered division of labour in modern societies these tensions have particular implications for women. As feminist researchers have pointed out, the literature suggest that women experience a distinctive tension between the dominance of monochronic or clock time and the polychronic or 'process time' (Davies 1989) which characterises the domestic sphere (Davies 1989; Glennie and Thrift 1996).

[P]rocess time means that the task itself defines the amount of time to be consumed, rather than a time limit or temporal demarcation being placed on the task. [...] [C]are work (whether it is carried out in the home or not) is characterised by short cycles that are frequently repeated and by the fact that it is *with difficulty* subsumed under strict clock time. (Davies 1989: 36, emphasis in original)

These observations are particularly pertinent to any understanding of the organisation of ward-based hospital nursing.

Time, space and the social organisation of nursing work on hospital wards

Ward-based nurses and support workers[2] are the only occupations on the hospital staff whose work is embedded in the temporal worlds of patients. They work in the spaces occupied by the sick and needy and they are guided by a practice ideology that emphasises the importance of a patient-centred approach, oriented to individual need. At the same time, however, most nurses deal with multiple patient assignments, and their work on the ward is embedded in a wider organisation, which is temporally and spatially complex. This makes it necessary to prioritise competing and often unpredictable patient needs and to co-ordinate these with the external timetables of the hospital and other specialists who come to the ward to attend to the patient.

The requirement to manage this kind of turbulence (Melia 1979) leads to the development of routines. All of the wards studied had an elementary routine to which all staff oriented and by which they monitored their work progress. Ward routines helped to ensure that the organisation of patient care did not conflict with the wider temporal structures of the hospital and that all patients received, at a minimum, a basic standard of provision (Allen 1996). Yet, while routines help nurses to manage their work, they are also constraining, creating a further obstacle to the provision of individually tailored care.

It is the requirement to manage this tension between the polychronic organisation of individualised care, the monochronic organisation of ward routines and the overall temporal structure of hospital organisation which constitutes the temporal perspective of hospital nurses and which is captured in various ways in the following extracts.

> I was talking to my student about it the other day. [...] I was discussing how he was doing and everything. [...] We were sort of saying that his care's fine what he's doing but I was saying he's not got a broad look. I said 'I have sort of a menu in my head'. I have like a time clock and

you're not consciously doing it but you're looking at the clock and you're thinking 'Yes at 10 o'clock such-and-such needs doing, and oh 11 o'clock such-and-such needs doing' and you just keep taking these bits of information and I think I slot them into my clock. (Interview – Senior nurse)

You usually do think 'Well I'd better get everybody washed by 11 o'clock or something at the latest. I'd better get most of the stuff out of the book done by such-and-such time'. I usually think that with things like organising transport and things like that because by 4 o'clock everything seems to close. You can't seem to get hold of anything. You try and do those because you think the late staff could be really busy, they might have a lot of discharges on the early you know, they might be trying to sort out all the admissions from [the admissions ward] so you usually think 'I'll try and get all So-and-so sorted out'. You know things like referring to the social worker. (Interview – Staff nurse)

They do a record-keeping day here and they say that there shouldn't be any diaries or anything like that. You should go on and you should look at your careplans and you know exactly what care to give to that patient. But I'm sorry in an ideal world, realistically if as soon as you walk on that ward and you start walking round looking at careplans the buzzers are going, the breakfasts arrive, people want a wash, they want to get out. You can't do it. You'd get half way down and then what? Somebody might have a colonoscopy booked for 10 o'clock and by the time you've got there it's too late and they've missed their enema that they should have had at 8 o'clock because you started at the other end instead of that end. (Interview – Staff nurse)

To a considerable extent, the organisation of nursing work and nurses' practical jurisdiction, that is their work content, arises from the need to balance these linked temporal tensions. In the following sections, I examine the impact of the temporal–spatial organisation of nursing work on the intra-occupational division of labour and nurses' boundary with medical and support staff.

Nursing's intra-occupational division of labour

Of all the occupational groups that comprise the hospital division of labour, it is only the nursing and support staff that provide 24-hour coverage, which is typically organised around a shift system. Within nursing culture, the 'handover' has a ritual significance (Zerubavel 1979a; Wolf 1988; Frankenberg 1992), marking the transference of responsibility from one shift to another. Possibly because caring – like women's work (Oakley 1974a,b) – is never done; nurses appear to derive a certain amount of job-satisfaction by accomplishing a pre-determined amount of work within the time-frame of a given shift. This was an unspoken rule on the wards studied: nurses clearly felt obliged to account for any failure to 'finish' the work.

> I think we all want to be super efficient. We all want to be super-nurse and make sure everything's done before the next [shift], because if you left something, it's an unsaid thing, but if you left something from the morning that you should have done in the morning or you think you should have done, you feel guilty all day. 'I'm sorry I haven't done that', 'Oh I haven't had chance to do that', 'Oh there looks a lot in this afternoon but there isn't really'. (Interview – Staff nurse)

Impersonality is central to any system of continuous coverage (Zerubavel 1979a). That any nurse can periodically interrupt continuity of patient coverage at the end of a shift is possible mainly because another person, defined as their functional equivalent, can take over their responsibilities. Historically, in the UK, when nurses in training were an integral part of the hospital labour force, the impersonality of nursing care provision was exacerbated further by the need to manage a transient student work force (Melia 1987; Proctor 1989; Davies 1995). Patient care was broken into a series of different tasks to be performed according to a set routine, thereby creating a series of pre-determined roles into which students could be slotted according to their stage of training. The corollary of organising work in this way, however, is that emphasis is given to the accomplishment of time-bounded physical caring *tasks* at the expense of the less visible *time* that is given to patients in order for them to discuss their needs and concerns or in assisting their return to independence. Moreover, responsibility for the work and standards of care is diluted amongst the team. In the context of widespread criticism about the impersonal nature of hospital care and against a tide of growing dissatisfaction with the organisation and content of nurses' work, new systems for organising nursing work have emerged aimed at promoting individualised patient care. Foremost amongst these is 'primary nursing'.[3]

'primary nursing' involves allocating 24-hour responsibility for each patient to a trained nurse, who plans, gives, supervises and evaluates individually tailored care, wherever possible with the active collaboration of the patients and their family. A premium is placed on the establishment of a close therapeutic relationship between the nurse and client. The primary nurse leads a team of 'associate' nurses who deliver care when the primary nurse cannot. Associate nurses are expected to administer the prescribed care rather than take diagnostic or prescriptive decisions.

One difficulty with the 'primary nursing' model, however, is that it is based on the assumption of a richly skilled nursing work force. In the UK certainly, research has shown that few hospitals have been able to implement it fully, most opting for a team nursing model (Mead and McGuire 1993). This was the case in the research locale. On the two wards studied, this entailed the creation of two teams – red and blue – comprising a mixture of qualified staff, support workers and students. Each team was led by a nurse, who assumed responsibility for the management and supervision of care. Patients were allocated to a team for the duration of their hospital admission in order to promote continuity. Responsibility for the co-ordination of overall ward activity fell to the senior nurses in both settings.

While the adoption of a system of team nursing was in many respects a pragmatic response to the realities of service provision – that is, an acknowledgement by nurse managers that the grade and skills mix on the ward did not permit the use of a 'primary nursing' model – its successful implementation was nevertheless impeded by the organisation of care on the wards. Owing to the spatial arrangement of patients and the polychronic nature of care, the staff found it impossible to limit their work activities to meeting the needs of those patients who were in 'their' team.

> The ward is all mixed you see, and when a blue patient says to you 'Can you take me to the toilet?', you can't very well say 'No you've got to ask the red person'. (Interview – SEN)

> Tanya [staff nurse] said that she liked team nursing – what she did not like was when she ended up 'bay nursing'. By this she meant when she went into one bay and ended up giving out bowls to all of the patients in the bay. She said that this happened often. She said you go into a bay and give out bowls to your patients and then all the others ask for

one – then you can't nurse as a team. She said that she did not like that. (Fieldnotes)

Jennifer sat at the nurses station – she said that she could not get used to the way of working of the ward – with the patients 'scattered all over the place'. 'I much prefer bay nursing' she said. She went on, 'How can you go into a bay and another patient asks you for something and you have to say sorry you're not in my team I'll get someone who is. It's much easier if all of your patients are in the same bay'. (Fieldnotes)

It was, in part, for these reasons that the nurses insisted on making sure they were aware of the detail and progress of *all* patients on the ward rather than concentrating solely on those in their teams.

Although team nursing is very much a watered-down version of the 'primary nursing' ideal, it nevertheless retains an emphasis on the centrality of the nurse–client relationship, which is commonly expressed in nursing parlance as 'knowing the patient'. Yet, team nursing (and 'primary nursing' for that matter) still has to be accomplished within a model of shift working and, within modern day healthcare systems, patient turnover is high. Despite the importance of handover and the nursing record as mechanisms for the maintenance of continuity, it was commonplace for nurses to express frustration at not 'knowing' the patients on their return from days off.

The specialist nurse came to the ward to see Mr Wilson. She stops to talk to Jane [senior nurse] at the nurses' station.

Specialist nurse: Mr Dobson?

Jane: Yes?

Specialist nurse: How is he?

Jane: Can you have a word with Jenny because this is my first day back. (Fieldnotes)

Auxiliary: She's poorly the lady in bed one bay five.

Staff nurse: I don't know these bay five patients on here. I'd feel a lot better when I've been on a couple of nights. (Fieldnotes)

Interestingly one of the ways in which nurses could be reminded about their knowledge of patients was by reference to their spatial location within the ward area.

HCA: Is it all right if Mrs Furnace has a bath?

Senior nurse: Errr [*closing her eyes struggling to think who the patient is*].

HCA: Bay two, bed three.

Senior nurse: Oh yes – yes that's all right.   (Fieldnotes)

Nurse 1: Mrs Toone – did she walk to the toilet or did she go on the chair? I can't remember.

Nurse 2: Mrs who?

Nurse 1: Bay four, second bed.   (Fieldnotes)

For the nurses in this study 'knowing the patient' did not seem to imply the level of intimacy suggested by some interpretations of nursing's 'therapeutic gaze' (e.g. May 1992). Rather it related to having up-to-date knowledge of the patient's progress and their relevant social circumstances. Nevertheless, despite this tempering of the professional vision, to not 'know' all aspects of care relating to one's patient was a threat to a nurse's professional identity and an important source of job dissatisfaction.

The nurse–doctor boundary

Biographies

Strauss *et al.* (1985) have directed attention to the importance of 'biographies' in any temporal analysis of organisations and they outline a range of biographies they believe may be included: technological biographies, life histories of individual occupations, different personal biographies of employees and clients, as well as the biography of the organisation itself and its sub-units. One feature of the temporal–spatial organisation of hospitals that is particularly pertinent to any discussion of the medical–nursing boundary is its status as a training institution. The day-to-day medical care on hospital wards is provided by doctors in training who rotate around the various specialities. As Zerubavel (1979a) observes, the shortness of medical staff placements often leads to a reversal of the normal relationships with nurses.

The ethnographic literature indicate that stable nursing staffs can exert considerable influence over transient doctors (Mumford 1970; Bucher and Stelling 1977; Myers 1979;

Roth and Douglas 1983; Haas and Shaffir 1987; Hughes 1988) and on both of the wards studied, the relative permanency of nurses augmented their influence. As well as being an important source of information on more mundane details such as the location of equipment, nurses were also the guardians of local protocols and aspects of clinical practice. For example, nurses frequently queried drug prescriptions if they were different from the standard medication regimes with which they were familiar and it was commonplace for doctors to seek nurses' advice about prescription details.

> *House officer:* Does he have dextrose saline at all or does it have to be normal saline?
>
> *Staff nurse:* [*Off-hand*] Whatever. Either. (Fieldnotes)

Nurses routinely requested or made suggestions about prescribing medication for patients. In the following extract the house officer has been called to seen an elderly female patient who has become distressed. It echoes the findings of other recent ethnographic research (Hughes 1988; Porter 1991) which indicates that much contemporary nurse–doctor interaction goes beyond the inter-professional game-playing described by Stein (1967).

> *Staff nurse:* What's she going to have for pain then? What about Pethidine IM? [intra-muscular]
> There is no answer.
>
> *Staff nurse:* No?
>
> *House officer:* I was going to give her Diamorphine but she says it makes her feel sick.
>
> [*The nurses are chatting casually. The doctor finishes writing in the patient's notes and goes to leave.*]
>
> *Staff nurse:* What are you doing?
>
> *House officer:* Well she's sleeping now isn't she.
>
> *Staff nurse:* But I don't want you going and then she wakes up again because you won't be happy if we bleep you again [...]
> The doctor stays and there is a discussion [...] about painkillers. The doctor has prescribed oral DF118.
> The doctor goes to leave again [...]
>
> *Staff nurse:* So are you going to put that IM if need be?
> The doctor is looking in the BNF [British National Formulary].
>
> *Staff nurse:* The dose is fifty.
>
> *Sister:* She's happy to have oral. She's feeling a lot better now and she's tired.

The doctor is still hesitating about what to prescribe.

Staff nurse: Just put stroke [forward slash] IM.

House officer: But the dose is fifty and the tablets are thirty to sixty milligrams.

Staff nurse: Yes but what I'm saying is they come in fifty milligram ampoules and so if you write 'stroke IM' and I give that then I'm within that range.

The doctor does as staff nurse suggests. (Fieldnotes)

The temporal–spatial organisation of medical and nursing work

Medical and nursing staff orbit along different trajectories, nurses on one location but through a 24-hour shift system, doctors around the physical geography of a hospital or a group of hospitals. This [...] 'time-space geography' of medicine and nursing [...] presents practical difficulties in maintaining effective information exchanges, and creates differences in patient care priorities. (Walby and Greenwell *et al*. 1994: 92)

To this one might also add: it creates different temporal perspectives, leads to a blurring of role boundaries and creates an emotional division of labour that can lead to disagreements about patient treatment.

Different temporal–spatial perspectives

The nurses and doctors in the study site had very different temporal–spatial perspectives. Nurses, as we have seen, had a strong orientation to the monochronic constraints of the organisation, which was not shared by doctors. A significant amount of nurses' energy was directed at organising the doctors to ensure that they had accomplished the work that they needed to do within a given time-frame.

Sister was trying to contact Dr Ross.

Sister: Right doctor Ross – where are you?

Physiotherapist: You love him really!

Sister: He knew Mr Williams was going to theatre and he's not organised an ECG, a chest X-ray or bloods. We've had to do it all this morning.

Physio: Oh shit! [*Puts hands over her mouth*]. Sorry!

[...]

PE: And there's no pre-med. (Fieldnotes)

16:45 – there are still some things that need doing by the doctors on the ward. The doctor's finish at five. Staff nurse bleeps Dr Black and tells him that he has some TTOs to do [prescribe tablets for patients to take home]. She also bleeps Dr Duncan and asks him if he's busy on the admissions ward. Presumably he says that he is because she offers to bring the TTOs to him so he can prescribe them as they need to be done by five so they can go to pharmacy. HCA goes down to the admissions ward with the TTOs and then takes them straight to pharmacy. (Fieldnotes)

Yet, although nurses were frequently concerned with organising the doctors, it was also the case that doctors faced other demands on their time and often had different priorities than the nurses (see also Annandale *et al.* 1999). As a number of authors have observed, the bleep system can become a focus for these tensions (Frankenburg 1992; Walby and Greenwell *et al.* 1994). On one of the wards studied I came across an 'untoward incidents' book in which the most commonly recorded 'incidents' related to doctors' failure to attend to patients.

We have been bleeping the doctors since 9:30 to resite cannulas, patients to see, Mrs McClean, Mr Cousins, Mrs Woodhouse. Doctor came to the ward at 13:00 hrs but then got called away. 14:00 hrs doctor has still not been to the ward. (Document)

The nurses' frustration was matched by that of the medical staff who complained about their work being continuously interrupted by nurses bleeping them.

'Right I start the ward round here and go round to every ward. I will be some time there whenever this will be depends on the patients on each ward. So don't bleep me again. Save all my jobs I will be there some time'. And it sometimes happens that it's hours and then they get worried or whatever I think they think you're sitting in the canteen – I don't know what they are thinking – but you get bleeped all the time. This particular Sunday that I am talking about I was more than fifty times bleeped. It really drives you mad. So I don't know. They should know that you're going round sometimes. (Interview – Senior house officer)

Although pressures of work are a contributory factor, these strains over the bleep are also a product of the different temporal perspectives of doctors and nurses and the divergent priorities to which these give rise. Ward nurses were typically concerned with the immediate needs of their patients whereas doctors had much wider concerns.

House Officer said that the nurses often got cross when the Warfarin and things like that didn't get done but that they ranked quite lowly in the doctor's priorities. (Fieldnotes)

House Officer: Haematology patients, Rheumatology patients,
Medical patients – they're all patients.　　　　　　(Fieldnotes)

Furthermore, whereas nursing coverage is provided 365 days
a year, full medical cover is only provided on weekdays
between 9 and 5. Outside of these hours medical care was provided by an on-call system. This could lead to contrasting definitions of what constituted emergency cover.

Staff nurse 1: I've got some jobs.

House officer: As long as it's only prescribing!

Staff nurse 1: Oh! [*Passing doctor a drug kardex*] She needs that written up and a new drug kardex.

House officer: She needs an additional drug kardex.

Staff nurse 1: But it needs re-writing.

House officer: I'm not re-writing kardexes.

Staff nurse 1: But it will need doing tomorrow. Are you on? I suppose
not. What should I say? You refused to do it?

House officer: No, that the locum on-call doesn't re-write kardexes.

Staff nurse 2: Well this is something you should take up with your
medical colleagues then. Make sure they re-write kardexes on Friday.

　　　　　　(Fieldnotes)

The dilemma for nurses was that their work was embedded in
the polychronic care needs of patients, which were at odds
with the monochronic scheduling of the hospital organisation.
Moreover, it was nurses who had to cope with distressed and/
or irate patients whose requirements were not being met.

Staff nurse: Do you want any painkillers? I know your painkillers
haven't been working but they've not been changed yet so do you
want some Coprox?

Patient: [*Very annoyed*] Haven't they changed them yet? I've been asking since 10 o'clock. I've been in agony all day. I've asked about five
different nurses.

Staff nurse: [*Sounds slightly indignant*] But it isn't us that change them
you see. It is the doctors.

Patient: I know that but they said they'd leave a note on it.

Staff nurse: They have but. Do you want a Coprox then?

Patient: I suppose I'd better hadn't I.　　　　　　(Fieldnotes)

One of the ways in which nurses managed these potential points
of inter-occupational strain was by informally undertaking

a range of activities that officially should have been carried out by the doctor. This boundary-blurring was extensive and led to nurses regularly breaking organisational policies. For example, nurses requested blood tests, prescribed additional intravenous fluids, made referrals to the dietician and 'prescribed' medications for symptom relief (for a more detailed analysis of nurses' boundary-blurring practices see Allen 1997; Allen and Lyne 1997).

> *DA*: What about ECGs?
>
> *Staff nurse*: We do ECGs but it's an extended role isn't it? Often you'll get a doctor and they'll say 'You have a patient with chest pain. Do an ECG'. If you turn round and say 'Well we can't', then they won't have an ECG whilst they're in pain because by the time the doctor's got on to the ward then it's gone. At the end of the day it's patients and their care. It's the patient's best interests really.   (Interview – Staff nurse)

> *Staff nurse*: Yes we shouldn't be doing that should we but again it needs doing. Especially when you've got other consultant's patients on the wards and you know for a fact that they need this blood test doing and they won't come on and the phlebotomist is saying 'Oh I did this yesterday', INR for example 'I did this yesterday on them. Does this need doing today?' and you say 'Well yes it does', so you sign it don't you? You know that they're not going to come on immediately and sign it for you and you also know you'll be battling all day to try and get them to take the blood because the phlebotomist didn't.   (Interview – Staff nurse)

As Mauksch (1966) observes 'the role of the nurse is profoundly affected by her obligation to represent continuity of time and space' (120).

The ecology of knowledge and the emotional division of labour

The temporal–spatial organisation of medical and nursing work positions doctors and nurses differently in relation to patients. Ward staff have continuous contact with patients, whereas doctors have only a fleeting acquaintance. Doctors depend on nurses to provide them with clinically relevant information about the patient's progress and this casts nurses in a potentially powerful position in relation to clinical decision making. As Anspach (1987, 1993) has observed, however, these temporal–spatial variations in the social organisation of nursing and medical work create different interpretative frameworks within which doctors and nurses perceive their patients (see also Goode 1994; Mueller 1997). Nurses typically perceive the patient in broad terms: their medical and care needs are placed alongside their social and psychological needs. Doctors, by contrast, have a narrower technological focus. And although, at one level, nurses do exert considerable power over clinical decisions through the information they provide to medical staff, ultimately the final decision rests with the doctor and this can cause conflict and ethical dilemmas (Zussman 1992; Mueller 1997; Chambliss 1997).

> We'd all arranged for [a patient] to go home and he was all ready, his family were here, we'd got all this back-up for him and they were quite happy for him to go home with a catheter in and then [registrar] did the round and said 'He's stopping. I don't want him to go home with his catheter in. Take it out. If he's OK over the weekend then he can go home'. And we thought 'Oh my God we've made all these arrange-ments'. So I said to Sister [...] I said 'He's not doing that. I'm sorry – he's not doing that at all'. So I said will you have a word with him because if I have a word with him I'll probably shout at him and he'll probably just laugh'. So she says 'Yes. OK I'll have a word'. So she told him she said, 'Look we've got a district nurse going in, his family are happy to keep the catheter in because he was incontinent at home and they couldn't go out anywhere because he was always incontinent and they were just happy that now they would be able to take him out and not have to worry and he won't worry either'. He wouldn't have it – 'No, no I'm sorry I'm not happy about it. He's stopping'. When actually [the consultant] had said he could go home this weekend and we told [the named nurse] and [the named nurse] just got really upset and she said 'That's it I'm going to have a go at him now. I don't care'. So [the named nurse] went and had a go at him and he ummed and arrhed and got a bit funny with her and got a bit shirty but she says 'This man has been looking forward to going home all day, his relatives have been so pleased to get him home'. And all [registrar] kept saying was 'Well he shouldn't really go home with his catheter in.' He's got some sort of valve disorder and this that and the other but we were saying 'They know the man's condition. They know that they'll probably not have long with him. They want to share all they can with him at the moment' – you know and he didn't like it but we got our own way. [...] But we've often said to him 'All right you care for the patients, but not like we do. You come and you say "Put them on so-and-so" you know you prescribe them different things, order different investigations, but we're the ones that make sure that they get carried out and give them care, we're the ones that see them every day'. (Interview – Staff nurse)

As this extract indicates the temporal–spatial organisation of medical and nursing work creates a distinctive emotional division of labour between medical and nursing staff. The continuous contact that nurses had with patients made it less easy for them to develop the detached concern (Lief and Fox 1963) of doctors. Frankenberg (1992) cites the case of Kushlick *et al.* (1976) who, in giving evidence to a government committee, suggested that carers should be categorised according to the amount of time they spent with the cared-for. He argued that knowledge should be shared in both directions so that those continuously responsible for life decisions should not only be listened to but also kept fully informed of technological advances. Such was the entrenched power of the medical profession, however, that Kushlick was assumed to be speaking in jest!

The Nurse – support worker boundary

Non-nursing duties?

The dominance of western societies by monochronic (male) time has had particular ramifications for nursing. As Davies (1989) observes, conventional time-use studies typically omit many of the ways in which women use time. Spending time with children and playing with them is not included, nor is the emotional labour women carry out in caring for family members. What is also absent is recognition that women frequently are engaged in several activities simultaneously.

It is easy to see how these general observations translate into practice for nurses. Against the escalating costs of health service provision, nursing labour has been increasingly subject to scrutiny in the search for cost-containment. One of the perennial difficulties for nurses, however, is that time and motion studies frequently employ a gendered lens.

> [T]ime generating and time giving activities have no place in the meaning cluster of quantity, measure, dates and deadlines, of calculability, abstract exchange value, efficiency and profit. They simply cannot feature in the analysis. (Adam 1995: 95)

Numerous studies have made recommendations for the more efficient use of nursing labour, and in so doing, they have revealed their fundamental misunderstanding of the way in which nursing work is organised (e.g. Ball and Goldstone 1987). For example, research published in 1996 by the Health Services Management Unit at Manchester University caused some disquiet amongst nurses when, in addressing the question, 'if we were designing the workforce today for tomorrow's health service, what would it look like?', it suggested the development of a 'generic worker' role in the health services (Health Services Management Unit 1996). The warrant for this view was evidence of the amount of time nurses spent on direct patient care which implied that time spent doing other kinds of work is inappropriate. Yet, much of nurses' work involves care management and co-ordination and although not direct care as such, it is an essential and skilled role. Moreover, because 'care' is embedded in social relationships it does not lend itself to a rationalisation of tasks. On both wards in the study site, nurses regularly performed duties that, to an outside observer, might be considered a waste of their skills and more appropriately delegated to support staff. The incorporation of mundane activities into the nursing role occurred at a number of levels.

The care needs of patients are often immediate and unpredictable. Caring for someone means giving 'time' to them and making them the centre of attention. Nurses often undertook relatively unskilled work simply because they happened to be on the spot at the time.

> *Sister:* If you happened to be there and the patient needs something then you do it for them however expensive you might be.
>
> (Fieldnotes)

At another level, because care is characterised by polychronic rather than monochronic time, it is oriented to context and involves doing many things at once (Oakley 1974a,b; Hochschild 1989). It was often expedient, therefore, for nurses to undertake apparently mundane work while carrying out other skilled nursing activities. For example, I observed that they tidied the patient bed areas as they updated their patients' charts at the end of the shift. Such 'housekeeping' could be construed as a misuse of nursing time by health service managers, but viewed from a caring perspective, not only was it pragmatic, it made a vital contribution to the maintenance of a safe environment for patients and was a way of 'making time' for patients in an otherwise turbulent work context. By embedding time-giving in routine tasks, moreover, the nurses were able to ensure that 'time' was equally distributed amongst the total patient population.

> *DA*: I've seen you go round with your trolley – tidying up at the beginning of a shift.
>
> *Sister*: But I use that as a way of finding out if there's a problem [...] I won't spend long with everybody because some don't need you. It's just a case of 'Hello how are you getting on? How many times have you passed your water?' [...] I will also like tidy things up as I go [...] I think if it was me, at least if somebody's coming round all the time if there's something that they want to ask they are going to eventually ask somebody. So you just make yourself available.   (Interview)

A further way in which mundane work was woven into the fabric of nursing care was when nurses undertook an observable routine task in order to structure another, more complex but invisible, activity. This was a strategy nurses frequently employed so as to manage an interactional encounter with patients or their family and put themselves in a position to build relationships in a fashion that was socially comfortable for all concerned.

> [J]ust to go round each patient, sit by them and chat to them all, it can put them on edge. If it's new staff and you can go in and do something and take the emphasis off that and see what's happening to them, they feel a little bit more relaxed. Rather than you sitting there and drilling them and seeing how they are. You know 'Open up to me. Tell me all your problems.' (Interview – Staff nurse)

To summarise then, it would have been utterly impractical to divest nurses of all mundane work and any attempt to do so ignores the complexities of nursing practice (Allen 2001a).

Hands-on care

A second element in the debates about the division of labour between nurses and support staff relates to nurses' involvement in hands-on care. In recent years, the importance of basic nursing has been resurrected in feminist inspired ideologies of nursing practice and this has led to an attempt to reintegrate hands-on care into the core nursing role. Yet, as we have seen, these developments within the profession have taken place against a backdrop of increasing economic scrutiny of health service provision. Despite the importance attached to physical tending by the profession itself, in real life nursing practice, patient needs have to be met with a mixture of qualified and unqualified staff, the ratio of which has been increasingly diluted by cost-conscious health services managers (Ranade 1994). In both of the wards studied, it was necessary for nurses to 'ration' their involvement in hands-on care (Allen 2001a) and, in the main, this appeared to be shaped by the temporal rhythms of the ward and patients.

During the week nurses had numerous demands on their time and this shaped the extent to which they were able to involve themselves in direct patient care (see also Annandale *et al.* 1999). Up until about 9 o'clock nurses worked alongside support staff assisting patients with washes and their breakfasts. Thereafter, however, as the monochronic temporal rhythms of the wider organisation gained momentum their energies were directed elsewhere.

> *Staff nurse*: Until about 09:30 you're with your patients doing the baths. That's when you get your patient contact. But then you have to leave the auxiliaries to finish off the baths because you have all the obs to do and the diary to sort out. You spend all your time sorting out the diary.   (Fieldnotes)

As Mauksch observes:

> The social fact and general expectation of continuous and obligatory physical presence in the midst of many transient specialists is likely to saddle the occupant of the resident position with the latent function of co-ordinating those who come and go. Merely by virtue of being present, the nurse is expected to keep order in the flow of traffic and in the sequence of events that are scheduled for the patient. (Mauksch 1966: 120)

I observed that nurses took the opportunity to undertake hands-on care work at the weekends when the wards were generally quieter and the demands of the co-ordinating role greatly reduced.

The temporal–spatial organisation of ward work shaped nurses' involvement in hands-on care in other ways. Because of the turbulence of the ward environment, the unpredictability of patient need and the threat of an emergency, nurses tried to organise their work so that they were available to flexibly deploy their skills should they be required. As a consequence, it was support staff that assisted patients in the bathrooms. For the majority of patients on the wards the bathrooms were the only truly private spaces in which staff and patients could interact, and as such, it seems to me that the spatial organisation of work had important implications for the emotional division of labour on the ward. In contrast to nursing's professional claims about their close therapeutic relationships with patients, in practice it was support staff who were best placed to give *time* to them.

In this section, I have described the ways in which the temporal–spatial organisation of ward work shaped nurses' involvement in hands-on care. Clearly, this was not the only factor. If the ward had been staffed by an all qualified workforce, rather than a mixture of qualified nurses and support staff, then the work may have been organised rather differently. However, whilst a long-held aspiration of certain segments within the occupation, an all-qualified nursing workforce remains just that. Given the economic realities of the health service, support workers of one form or another seem likely to remain.

The support worker role?

In this final section, I want to explore how the biographies of support staff interacted with the temporal–spatial organisation of ward work and the implications that this had for the nurse–support worker boundary.

Biographies
On both wards, work was rooted in social relationships and allocated on the basis of trust and personal knowledge of staff skills rather than formal credentials. In their accounts of their work practices the staff frequently appealed to 'experience'. By this, they were referring to experience of work at the hospital as well as personal life experience. The preference for mature

auxiliaries which was expressed by one ward sister, appeared to be widely endorsed by both ward staffs and this shaped the division of labour in important ways.

I know Betty and I have noticed, sometimes with the older men they don't like to deal with them. Only because they're young girls and they'll send us in and we – like if you've a sheath to put on or things like that – things like that don't bother Betty and I at all but I can understand why they might get a little embarrassed about it and we can laugh it off. Because they get embarrassed with young nurses dealing with them but they tend not to with older women. I don't know why. Maybe because we're older and they seem more relaxed with us. So they'll say to us 'Go and put us a sheath on him' and you don't mind because you're older. And we'll say 'Oh aye – sending for Majorie Proops again', and we'll have a laugh about it. But we do find it easier than the youngsters. And I think that's understandable, I understand that I really do and I think that's nice that they can do that with us. (Interview – HCA)

[L]ike dealing with bereaved relatives, some people might think that she [HCA] shouldn't get involved, that it should be the staff nurses, but I think that she's had a lot more life experience than me and you know she perhaps could talk to them more. So I think get involved. (Fieldnotes – Staff nurse)

Routines
The processes of routinisation on both wards meant that the work of nursing and support staff was clearly differentiated in time and space.

We do our work and the nurses do theirs. (Fieldnotes – Auxiliary)

Even when the nurses and support staff worked together washing patients and preparing them for breakfast they tended to different patients. Nurses stayed in the main ward areas from where their skills could be utilised if required, whereas the auxiliaries would work in the bathrooms. If no support staff were on duty then the chances of their work being overlooked was high.

These arrangements afforded the support workers considerable freedom in the performance of patient care. Indeed, it was frequently the case that the nursing gaze had to be filtered through the interpretative lens of support staff (Allen 2001a, for a comparison, see also Chapter 7, this volume). Consonant with findings elsewhere in the literature (Strauss *et al.* 1964;

Scheff 1961; Mechanic 1961; Towell 1975) this put them in a powerful position from where they were able to exercise indirect control over nursing and medical decisions. Yet, although this state of affairs contravened the formal organisational plan – in which remuneration for support staff was based on the assumption that they worked under constant supervision on the wards – where relationships were established these arrangements had advantages for both parties. Nurses appreciated working with support staff that could be trusted to work without supervision and the support staff valued the autonomy these arrangements afforded them.

> *Staff nurse*: Last night was awful. We had a bank auxiliary and she was useless. She just sat here at the desk all night. We didn't stop. Whereas tonight we've got two auxiliaries on and they're both really good so we can just leave them to get on with their work whereas last night you couldn't. I was doing IVs at 2 o'clock.   (Fieldnotes)

> Whether it's because I'm older I don't know because I am the oldest on the ward. I don't know but they let me do most things and they trust me to do most things and I try to respect that – that they give me that sort of responsibility but I have worked on one particular ward where they didn't let you even empty catheters which to me is. I can't understand why an auxiliary wouldn't be able to empty a catheter but I have heard that there are wards like that but I can't say on that on here. They let me do a lot of things. I mean maybe I shouldn't be doing them I don't know but if they can trust me to do that then that's fine. (Interview – HCA)

Conclusions

In this chapter, I have investigated how the temporal–spatial ordering of the hospital setting shaped the everyday work of ward nurses. I have argued that at its most fundamental level, nursing work involves mediating the polychronic temporal care needs of patients with the monochronic organisation of the hospital and I have described the tensions to which this gives rise. For example, we have seen how the need for care is not constrained by time or space and that amongst nurses this open-endedness creates a strong sense of work norms to be completed within particular time-frames. We have also seen how the temporal–spatial organisation of ward work made it difficult to implement team-nursing and for nurses to 'know' the patient.

In respect of the medical–nursing interface, I have shown how the experiential biographies of nursing and medical staff intersected to afford nurses' influence over clinical decision-making and how the different temporal–spatial organisation of their work led to nurses informally undertaking doctors' activities. In addition, I have argued that doctors and nurses inhabit different temporal–spatial worlds *vis-à-vis* the patient and this can create disagreements about treatment decisions.

Time and space also shape the emotional division of labour between nurses and support staff. Because of their vital coordinating role, nurses had to ration their involvement in hands-on care and, as a consequence, their 'knowing' of the patient had to be filtered through the interpretations of auxiliaries and HCAs. I have argued that contrary to their official job descriptions, support staff, were given considerable autonomy and were allocated work according to their experience rather than their credentials.

Taken as a whole these findings indicate that the real life work of hospital nurses is rather different from the kinds of claims which are made by some leaders of the profession and also the official organisational job descriptions. As such, there is nothing extraordinary about these findings. Organisational scholars have long recognised that everyday workplace reality is more complex than conventional wisdom allows. For the most part, however, we have had to be content with broad descriptions to capture this state of affairs – such as the 'negotiated order' (Strauss *et al.* 1985) or 'fuzzy workplace reality' (Abbott 1988) – less attention has been given to delineating in a systematic fashion those features of the work environment which shape the routine organisation of work and their effects. The findings explicated in this chapter indicate that the roles and responsibilities in the healthcare division of labour appear to be constituted, at least in part, by their location in time and space. Indeed one could go so far as to suggest that the division of labour on the hospital ward reflects a temporal–spatial jurisdiction rather than an occupational jurisdiction and that, for analytic purposes, it might be useful to make a distinction between the two.

3 Perceptions of teamwork in acute medical wards

Sherrill Snelgrove and David Hughes

Introduction

This chapter is concerned with the reality of teamwork for doctors and nurses working in the contemporary (National Health Service) NHS. Viewed from the perspective of the division of labour, teamwork is only one of several possible ways of organising relations between the specialists who contribute to the production of a service or commodity. However, the 'team' appears to be supplanting other modes of organisation, such as the bureaucratic hierarchy or collegial relations between independent professionals, as the favoured mode of delivering much of the work of healthcare. For this reason, and because modes of organisation, such as team, hierarchy or collegial relations, shape the experience of joint working, teamwork warrants study as an important aspect of the division of labour.

Although teamwork is often seen as a prerequisite for good practice in healthcare, the concept remains something of an enigma for social scientists. The language of 'team' is applied to a variety of working arrangements, encompassing a multiplicity of actors, in a range of settings. Teams may be formed around specialisms, professions and/or physical locales. They can be based on a single profession or formed on multi-disciplinary lines. Teams have varying degrees of permanency, can be organised in diverse ways and have different cultures and inter-personal dynamics. Some teams comprise loose groupings of people working towards a common purpose in a shared locale but never having formal meetings. Others are made up of persons who work in different areas but who attend pre-arranged meetings to conduct team business. Moreover, some areas, such as mental health and care of older people, have a much longer tradition of multi-disciplinary teamwork than others. Yet, alongside this diversity, there is a body of common-sense understandings about teamwork – an idealised version of team – that many people appear to share. Team members communicate and work together closely. Teams involve a flattening of hierarchies. Team working is co-operative and largely consensual. The high-perceived value of teamwork in health policy and practitioner circles appears to rest on a number of factors. It is partly about harnessing the different skills and competencies of the different health occupations to maximise the benefits for patient care, and improve co-ordination and inter-agency working. A number of commentators on the contemporary NHS sketch out an optimistic picture of professionals working as partners to provide improved patient care (Rowe 1996; Cott 1998). It has been argued that teamwork produces better care by reducing costs, benefiting the motivation and mental health of staff, and promoting the flexible use of knowledge and skills (Feiger and Schmitt 1979; Knaus *et al.* 1986; Firth-Cozens 1998; Macy and Izumi 1993; Ovretveit *et al.* 1997). This has been carried across into the policy discourse. One recent exemplification is the Department of Health (1998b) White Paper, '*A First Class Service*', which makes an explicit case for increased inter-professional collaboration. Another is the Government's current *NHS Plan*, which states that: 'Throughout the NHS the old hierarchical ways of working are giving way to more flexible team working between different clinical professionals' (NHS 2000: 9.2). The *NHS Plan* is sprinkled with positive references to the 'clinical teams' and 'primary health care teams' that will deliver improved care. The new arrangements are contrasted with the previous internal market system, and the associated 'market ethos [which] undermined teamwork between professionals and organisations vital to patient-centred care' (NHS 2000: 6.3).

Away from the policy rhetoric, many commentators argue that teamwork has emerged as a way of managing one of the main obstacles to inter-professional working – the problem of medical dominance. This is seen as a particular difficulty at the interface of health and social care, where relations between professionals from different disciplinary backgrounds have often been problematic. It has been suggested that teamwork attenuates the effect of traditional professional hierarchies and provides a framework for joint working that is acceptable to all the participants (Dingwall 1980). The greater emphasis on cross-disciplinary working is also related to the increased recognition of the importance of social aspects of care which has developed in parallel with expanded definitions of health and improved knowledge of social causes of ill health. And lastly, it fits well with the professionalising projects of some of the less well-rewarded occupations making up the healthcare division of labour, especially nursing.

Social scientists have also drawn attention to certain more problematic aspects of teams and teamwork. Rather than seeing teamwork as a product of shared conceptions of collegiality and equality, some have suggested that it may mean different things to different team members. Thus, teamwork may be seen as a (fragile) practical accomplishment emerging from the micro-political struggles of team members with different agendas and degrees of power (Dingwall 1980; Griffiths 1997), or even as a political rhetoric employed by different healthcare professionals for varying purposes (Griffiths and Hughes 1994). The suggestion here is that the language of 'team' has become part of a new orthodoxy to which many organisations pay lip service, even when there is little change in underlying patterns of behaviour.

Whilst there is a large literature on the benefits of teamwork, supporting research evidence is scarce (Zwarenstein and Reeves 2000). Certainly, there is plenty of potential for teams to get it wrong, and not all teams are effective (Firth-Cozens 1998). In the healthcare field, the individuals who staff multidisciplinary teams are drawn from occupational groups whose past relations have often been shaped by tribalism and competing interests (Strong and Robinson 1990). The recent Bristol Royal Infirmary Inquiry (Kennedy 2001), as well as several other high profile cases involving medical errors that went uncorrected by members of the healthcare team, indicate that the existence of 'teams' may in itself do little to counter self-protective professional practices. This is partly because teams in the healthcare domain often depart radically from the conventional understandings of the team concept:

[The consultants] saw these as their teams, which they led. They were not part of the team other than as leaders. Also the teams were teams of 'like professionals' [...] they were not cross-specialty or multi-disciplinary, and they were profoundly hierarchical. (Kennedy 2001: 15.8)

The doctor–nurse relationship is one of the most discussed and critiqued forms of 'teamwork' operating within Western healthcare systems (Wicks 1998). Social scientists have long observed that the relationship is rooted in a hierarchical division of labour and knowledge, in which inequalities of power are compounded by gender inequalities (Etzioni 1969; Freidson 1970a; Witz 1992). In the view of most early commentators, any influence exerted by nurses on doctors' decision making worked at the informal level. Thus, Stein (1967) described how newly qualified doctors took their cues from experienced nurses in a ritualised 'game', which enabled doctors to maintain a public face of authority while implicitly acknowledging nurses' superior hands-on knowledge. This picture of hierarchical relations, softened by a measure of covert influence by nurses who remained deferent to doctors, would seem to fly in the face of characteristics such as equality and collegiality that are required for successful teamwork.

Recent studies suggest that this traditional model is being eroded as the doctor/nurse relationship evolves in somewhat divergent ways in different healthcare settings. This can be linked to various influences including the changing 'knowledge contexts' of nursing (Svensson 1996), work pressures that lead nurses to cross traditional role boundaries (Allen 1997), and nurses' increased access to higher education and specialist courses (Snelgrove and Hughes 2000). It remains unclear how far such factors have a general impact, in terms of overturning the entrenched attitudes that have made the doctor–nurse relationship so unequal in the past. The growth of a team approach to healthcare, combined with increasing opportunities for nurses to develop autonomous professional practice, seems likely to accelerate the change process. This chapter addresses these issues by investigating understandings of teamwork as seen by hospital doctors and nurses working in general medicine. Teamwork was only one aspect of the wider study on the changing division of labour between medicine and nursing, and this chapter is based on a subset of our interview data.

The research

Data were obtained from interviews with samples of nursing and medical staff in three district general hospitals. The samples were randomly selected from the staffing lists of all medical wards, but were stratified to preserve the relative proportions of doctors and nurses working in the three hospitals. As nurses were a bigger staff group than doctors, it was decided to approach a 50 per cent sample of doctors and a 35 per cent sample of nurses. The resultant lists of staff to be approached for interview consisted of 27 doctors and 50 nurses. The nurses were all qualified RGNs (Registered General Nurse) or SENs (State Enrolled Nurse). The grades of the doctors ranged from junior house officer to senior registrar. The response rate was approximately 70 per cent, and 20 doctors and 39 nurses were interviewed in their place of work over a period of about four months. The interviews were divided between four researchers, two of whom were nurse lecturers.

A semi-structured interview guide was developed incorporating questions derived from the academic literature on interprofessional relationships and the 'doctor/nurse game'. These questions were supplemented by additional probes in areas where subjects offered more extended accounts. The interviews lasted between 45 and 60 minutes each, and were tape-recorded and subsequently transcribed. Transcriptions of interviews were analysed by identifying, ordering and coding relevant themes. Since many of the elements of the interview guide were derived from the existing literature, we make no claim that this is a wholly inductive approach. Indeed, one may suggest that such a purist approach is unrealistic even in a so-called 'grounded theory' study. However, we considered it important to engage seriously with the emerging data, so that novel findings were not overlooked. Much time was spent examining the transcripts for negative evidence and inconsistent or contradictory statements.

Research interviews take a variety of forms, ranging from the unstructured 'depth' interviews characteristic of phenomenological studies through to structured interviews where closed questions are used. We opted for semi-structured interviews to try to ensure uniformity of coverage across cases and the different interviewers. It was hoped that this approach would enable us to explore the themes that the literature had suggested were important, while also allowing the respondents space to contribute new insights.

Different formulations of 'team' and teamwork

Almost all the doctors and nurses interviewed espoused support for teamwork, but there were interesting differences in the way the two groups used the concept. Not only did doctors and nurses have different perceptions of the meaning of teamwork, but reference was made to different versions of 'team', which featured differently in doctors' and nurses' accounts.

Both groups sometimes used the term 'team' to describe working relations with colleagues from their own discipline. They used team to refer to the 'nursing team', in the sense of the informal workgroup of ward nurses. Respondents also spoke of 'team nursing', used as a shorthand term for the new patterns of working that had been introduced in some clinical settings.

> Lots of differences in practice since I started training such as nursing models, primary nursing, the nursing process, team nursing. We practice team nursing on this ward. Roper/Logan/Tierney is the model we use. (Staff nurse)

For rank-and-file nurses, the creation of teams of this kind had changed relationships with both senior nurses and doctors. It brought new ways of working in which individual nurses assumed responsibility for individual patients and might be required to communicate information about those patients directly to doctors, rather than – as in the past – using a senior nurse as an intermediary. Given this usage of the term, the existence of 'teams' was not necessarily something that brought the two occupations together, and might in some accounts be used to point to their different occupational identities and roles.

> Also there are two different teams of professions. The docs are there to diagnose the patient's illness; we're there to nurse the patient through the illness – the nursing team. (Sister)

If you're giving nursing care, that's not a medical decision; it's a nursing decision made with other members of the nursing team. (Charge nurse)

The constitution of a team defines the in-group but also serves to erect a barrier between members and non-members, and some nurses appeared to understand teamwork mainly in terms of informal workgroups of nurses and health care assistants (HCAs), which did not include doctors.

The interviews also contained references to two kinds of team that spanned disciplines. These might be described as the 'nurse/doctor care team' and the 'multi-disciplinary team'. The nurse–doctor care team is our gloss for the way many respondents used 'team' and 'teamwork' to describe everyday patterns of working between disciplinary colleagues in the main clinical areas. As mentioned above, 'team' might sometimes be used only to refer to the ward nurses, but on other occasions the focus was widened to include doctors, involved with nurses in ongoing, informal work activities. Here, the 'team' is the group of colleagues, including both doctors and nurses, who interact in the course of getting through the work. It provides the context in which the interface between the medical treatment and nursing care of the patient is negotiated.

Elsewhere, respondents talked of 'multi-disciplinary teams' as formally constituted teams that had been set up in some clinical areas to assist decision making on matters such as discharge planning. These teams held regular meetings, which took place weekly on many of the medical wards in the study. The team members typically comprised physiotherapists, social workers, district nurses and doctors, although the latter might not always attend. The focus of most multi-disciplinary teams was on discharge planning and other social concerns, such as liaison with relatives and outside agencies, rather than diagnosis and treatment.

The value of teamwork

Many doctors and nurses claimed to detect a move towards greater equality and away from traditional hierarchical relations. In their general statements, both groups constructed an idealised image of teamwork based on flattened hierarchies and greater opportunities for dialogue and shared participation in decision making. These accounts often included mention of the benefits that teamwork brought in terms of improved treatment and care of patients, and a better understanding of the work roles of other team members. For example, a senior house officer commented:

> Yes, working as a team. Each part is equally important depending on what specialty you are talking about. I think the 'physio' knows what we're doing, we know what they are doing – nice to know someone from all angles.

Both doctors and nurses pointed to a connection between more equal inter-professional relationships and better patient care.

> Yes, And I think that's very healthy. I think that if anyone thinks their decisions shouldn't be challenged then you'd end up with a very dull and staid way of doing things. It's actually quite good to create an environment where everybody feels they can contribute. It's good for the patient; it's good for the junior staff because everybody feels they are being listened to. (Registrar)

> We're all part of the same team with a common goal, which is to help the patient. It's better for the patient, working together. (Senior staff nurse)

Many nurses, in particular, went on to suggest that teamwork offered increased opportunities for shared decision making. Interestingly, this was not usually presented as following from joint deliberations between professionals possessing common expertise in a shared body of knowledge, but rather as an aspect of a division of labour. Thus, most respondents constructed an image of joint working by professionals who make different and complementary contributions to the care process.

> Partnership. The nurse listens to the doctor and the doctor listens to the nurse. I see the nurse's role as far more important. It's hit home to me that the nurse is the person who [...] who's there all the time: the doctor isn't. So if there's a cause for concern, it needs to be brought to the attention of the doctor. That's why I think it's a partnership. They help each other. (Staff nurse)

One difficulty in interpreting much of our data is that accounts that may at first sight seem to reflect traditional patterns of doctor/nurse interaction also fit well with a new feminist-inspired version of nursing practice (see also Chapter 1, this volume). The respondent above describes the nursing contribution to this 'partnership' in terms of activities that are well-documented in studies carried out over the past forty years or more. It was not based on control over advanced technologies or new areas for nurse decision-making, but on a close familiarity with the patient's clinical, personal and social circumstances that arises from continuity of care and other long-standing features of the hospital division of labour (Mauksch 1965; Zerubavel 1979b; Tellis-Nayak and Tellis-Nayak 1984). However, it is precisely the close and individualised nature of nursing care that has been taken up by the 'new nursing' and in associated ideas about holistic practice. Phrases such as 'brought to the attention of the doctor', may from this standpoint simply indicate a recognition of the different skills and spatial organisation of medical and nursing work, without implying that difference means hierarchy (see also Chapter 2, this volume). But this division of labour can also be formulated in just those terms, with nurses cast in the role of doctor's assistant. As was noted in Chapter 1, different work priorities may be formulated in terms of a social construction of skills, which values the technical above the general, and helps to perpetuate existing status hierarchies (Phillips and Taylor 1980; Davies and Rosser 1986; Davies 1995).

Sites for shared decision-making

Two points that emerged from an analysis of our interviews with nurses were first, that general statements about increased opportunities for shared decision-making were not always supported by credible examples of real decisions, and second, that most examples of 'joint decision making' that were cited related to discharge planning and social aspects of care.

> My decision making can be split into two areas. I can split the decisions that I make as far as the nursing practice goes, as related to patients, and the other half then is joint decisions with medical colleagues as regards patients' social circumstances, pulling social workers in, OTs (Occupational Therapist) in. (Staff nurse)

> In my team we say, 'Look, we think the patient should go home on Wednesday, is that okay for you? Usually they say 'Yes'. If they say 'No'

we listen to why they said 'No'. But it doesn't happen all the time. Eighty per cent of the time we find out if they have a problem or not. They come up to us and say 'Look we're going to have problems, we didn't send the woman home'. And we say 'That's fine by us'. Often we've said, 'Discharge home tomorrow', and we've come back the next day to find the patient's still there. So we ask what happened and they say: 'Oh we couldn't send them home because she had family problems, or she became breathless again' [...] It is not an area of conflict. (Senior house officer)

As the extract above suggests, such matters might figure in everyday ward interactions, and increasingly such decisions were formalised in meetings of the new multi-disciplinary teams. There are a few examples in our data where nurses shared other kinds of consequential decisions in informal interactions with doctors on the ward. Just as reported by Svensson (1996), nurses appeared generally satisfied with relations with medical colleagues, and presented their communications as open and frank, but they recognised that they were not equal partners. The picture that emerges is of doctors listening and taking account of what nurses say, but stopping short of inviting their full participation in decision-making. One area mentioned by several respondents in this context was ward rounds.

[O]n ward rounds you find consultants asking you social circumstances, who they live with, are they in nursing homes, do they have family, do they have back-up support – which the doctor doesn't know. So they get that information from us. (Sister)

The many references made to the multi-disciplinary team as one of the main arenas for shared decision making, raises the question of whether certain forms of 'more equal' interaction centred on meetings of this kind. Both nurses and doctors mentioned the low visibility of hierarchy in these team meetings, as compared with the version of teamwork enacted in ordinary work on the wards. Thus, a senior house officer, referring to a recently established multi-disciplinary team, noted that the 'equal weighting' given to different team members was not a 'general' phenomenon.

More of each exploring a particular point of view – each person's role is equally important but is a different role – a team effort. You sit down and make it a definite role everyone is given equal weighting. Probably this isn't done enough in general terms.

Another doctor reported:

> One of the great things about one particular job that I did was we
> would have [a neurological hospital in London] a weekly meeting
> which was a multi-disciplinary team meeting which included lots of
> physios, nurses, speech therapists, junior doctors and consultants and
> every patient would be talked about by each of the people there. Their
> ideas pooled and more business was done at that meeting every week
> than is done in five or six ward rounds at this hospital this hospital suf-
> fers for the lack of it I think. (Registrar)

Nurses too pointed to the multi-disciplinary team as an important vehicle for change in the nature of inter-professional
relationships:

> I think team. It's a more of a team. I think perhaps – the only other thing
> I can think of mainly has changed is with these multi-disciplinary
> teams. I think its far more involved with the nurses – I mean at ward
> level and the social workers and the doctors as well are involved in it.
> (Staff nurse)

> The nurse knows more about the background and social problems of
> the patient. There's far more dealings with multi-disciplinary teams,
> social workers, OTs. So that enables the nurse to get more of a back-
> ground to the patient, and certainly the doctors use that, they are very
> receptive to that information. (Staff nurse)

Most formal team meetings focused on discharge, rehabilita-
tion and social aspects of patient care. In these hospital settings the social dimension of illness was strongly recognised,
but the organisation of this aspect of patient care rested mainly
with the nurses and other paramedical professions. Many
nurses appeared to see their *de facto* responsibility for this
social domain as promoting a more autonomous nursing role,
and many doctors seemed only too willing to pass this work
across to nurses (see also Snelgrove and Hughes 2000).

Constructing domains of competence

The distinction between technical/physiological intervention,
on the one hand, and basic care and the management of the
social dimension, on the other hand, was central to most doctors' and some nurses' accounts of the division of labour within
teams. Doctors tended to locate their own work entirely within

the first category and that of nurses mainly in the second. By using a discourse that formulates expert technical activities as the core 'medical' work, they relegated other aspects of care to a secondary level.

In the first instance the decision making is almost entirely medical: you're using your medical skills to assess whether a patient is very ill, not very ill or not particularly unwell, and what you then do is very much gauged by your initial clinical impression [...] But then after that emergency situation other needs of the patient become more prominent: the need to assess their background, what their social circumstances are like, whether they have a supportive family, whether they're able to take certain forms of medication you think they may need. And there are many other factors that come in to how you treat a patient, but I think you can divide it into the emergency situation when decisions are almost exclusively medical and decisions about the broader patient's ongoing care. (Registrar)

In terms of deciding when a patient goes home and what their social circumstances are we almost hand those problems over to nursing staff because they are far more in touch with the social workers, the occupational therapists. So there's almost two phases, particularly in the elderly, where you have a patient coming in and the doctors have to be heavily involved initially getting the patient over their acute illness. If they are unable to go home straight away than it's the nursing staff that take responsibility for the ongoing physio-care, the dietician becoming involved, the social services going out and doing a home visit. So they are really vitally important from that point of view. (Registrar)

I think patients are looked after by the nurses and almost everything is done by them, and we only do the complicated stuff they can't do. And we advise them what we think is going on, how we should treat them, and we give specific directives to them. But the day-to-day things are done by them and they do a lot more patient counselling than us. (Senior house officer)

This primary division between core 'medical' work and care/support work provides a basis for other distinctions, such as that between the management of the patient and the disease on the one hand, and the care of the patient 'as a person' on the other hand. In several interviews the doctor is portrayed as a specialist whose role is to concentrate on the 'medical aspect' of the case, while the nurse is a generalist responsible for 'doing for' the person, and dealing with a variety of personal needs and problems.

As a doctor I am in charge of the patient, you know this relates to the traditional way of medical care, where I'm responsible for his management and for the management of his disease. For him or her as a person [...] nurses of course they are around to do for, they care for the patient as-well, together with me.

We just see the medical aspect of it but the nurses are more involved with other aspects of it as well. I think there is a better bond with the patients – the nurses rather than the doctors. We just come along and probably tell the nurses. (Senior house officer)

Most nurses recognise this divide, yet regard it with a degree of ambivalence. Certainly many wish to claim the social domain, as well as basic patient care work, as nursing territory.

I feel that the social care of the patient is the nurse's. The home care, circumstances when they'll be discharged, psychological care – if they feel they need more input psychologically. But you have to go to the doctor for referral or anything really. [...] and the basic nursing care – the bedbath, pressure areas, hydration – anything like that is nursing really. (Staff nurse)

Speaking to the relatives about everyday care of the patient, because we tell them about the patient. Maybe that's a possessiveness. I think the patient is ours. That's caring [...] I don't mind them [doctors] interfering, but they're our territory. They've got their model as well [...] We've got our model – caring model. (Staff nurse)

However, some nurses emphasised that they also possessed significant clinical skills. There is a long history of nurses acquiring *de facto* clinical skills via experience and observation, but recent changes in training and the emergence of a plethora of specialist roles mean that many now acquire these competencies through formal as well as informal pathways. Consequently, there was a significant group of nurses who, on the basis of training or experiential knowledge, asserted that teamwork should mean that they had a voice in some decisions within the technical/physiological domain. Nurses taking this stance rarely claimed full parity with medics in areas like diagnosis or treatment planning, but said that they wanted to be able to express a view, to pass on relevant information and, if necessary, to challenge decisions they believed to be mistaken.

Int: How acceptable is it for nurses to give doctors advice on clinical practice?

R: Very acceptable, particularly in places like coronary care where I worked. It used to be said that the nurses would do an ECG before the doctors turned around and said, 'What do you think this is and do you agree with it?' But like in coronary care if you're working in an area, a specialist area, like here with dermatology, we see these conditions, we see how they respond, when they don't respond. I mean we've got a wealth of information that we can provide.

Int: Have you offered advice?

R: Yes, it's received well by newly qualified house officers.

Int: Given advice to more senior doctors?

R: If I felt it was appropriate.

Int: Was it well received?

R: Yes. (Charge nurse)

I will openly challenge, especially if I have some alternative suggestion. (Staff nurse)

Expertise in specialist practice is an important lever for nurses seeking to augment their occupational position, but it may be difficult to balance greater engagement with the technical domain against support for nursing's caring model. Those who become experts in specialist roles risk the charge that they are undermining the more holistic version of nursing care associated with the 'new nursing' (see also Chapter 5, this volume). A number of doctors made positive statements about the increasing competence of nurses resulting from better training, as well as the value of experience.

Nurses know more, yes. It makes it a lot easier for us because they know more. They take away a lot of the care burden. For example if somebody comes in having diarrhoea the nurse knows exactly what to do: put the person in a cubicle and barrier-nurse the patient. They know when to send the specimens off. We don't have to bother to do all of that [...] They are just better trained. They know more. It helps everybody. It's good. It helps the patient; it helps us. (Senior house officer)

Many nurses are so experienced they can tell you: 'I think this is happening now, he's got left ventricular failure. That's why, he's got a history of this and I've seen it all before'. You tend to respect those kinds of observations, because they've been made with years of experience. (Senior house officer)

Some doctors recognise that an expanded role for nurses eases the burden falling on them by allowing the delegation of tasks, but increased involvement in the technical domain also puts nurses in a position where they can evaluate doctors' practice and offer advice with some credibility. Many doctors appeared ambivalent about the advice-giving role of nurses in relation to mainstream diagnosis and treatment planning. Where advice was accepted, this tended to be a conditional acceptance based on the characteristics of particular nurses or the needs of particular situations, rather than on shared technical expertise based on systematic training. Some doctors suggested that nurses' involvement in clinical decisions was problematic because their knowledge was variable and contingent on experience. While the basic competence of medical colleagues might be assumed until contrary evidence was forthcoming, the degree of competence of nurses was presented as being unpredictable.

> Equally there are other nurses – I don't think there's any difference in the knowledge of these two nurses – but they ring you up and you go there and it's an absolute waste of time. And you learn to recognise that as you stay in a place a long time. What I also feel is that too much knowledge is a bad thing. Especially when you are not entirely familiar with the whole practice of medicine. Some things you can suggest, and I always resent nurses who suggest particular treatment, particularly to junior doctors and who bully them into carrying it out. (Senior house officer)

> Well if the advice is stupid then it is not welcome, but if it's constructive, then yes. I was giving this drug to a patient and this patient had come in with other problems, problems with the heart and chest, but he also had porphyria – which is not really an active disease, his type of porphyria. But there are a lot of drugs counter-indicated there. Now I didn't know this chap had porphryia. He didn't tell me he had it. When the nurses' records had come around before the doctors' records, this nurse rang me and said, 'You know, you've prescribed him this drug but this chap has porphyria'. And I said 'hold it', and it's totally appropriate. Now I was thankful to her, she told me about it. It's extremely useful.[4] (Senior house officer)

Thus, many doctors appeared to approach nurses' advice with a degree of organised scepticism: it was presented as something that might well be of value, but which was often inaccurate or misleading because of an incomplete understanding of medical science. This could result in a mindset in which doctors were willing to acknowledge an advice-giving role for nurses, but wanted to set clear limits on where advice would end.

I think, yes, as long as its limited to being an advisory role, and nurses should definitely learn not to get a bee in their bonnet if their advice is not taken because I think that is what happens. If advice is given and it is not taken up, there are recriminations from that, which I think – they should always understand that advice is advice but they do not have the ultimate responsibility. (Senior house officer)

At the extreme, some doctors denied that there was any role for nurses in diagnosis, which they regarded as a technical task requiring core medical skills not possessed by the other group.

I can't see how a nurse would be able to help the diagnosis because that is entirely my specialty. I am thinking now about what I see inside an endoscopy. I would ask her probably about how to handle the endo-scope, but in the end what I see and what I decide on is entirely mine. She would probably be no help there. (Senior house officer)

Can teams co-exist with hierarchy?

It is evident from many of the data extracts in the previous section that doctors do not see nurses as equal partners, and that many nurses accept the reality of this situation. Although both occupational groups espouse support for teamwork, they have rather different understandings of what this means. Doctors generally present teamwork in terms of a division of labour between team members who bring different and com-plementary skills to the patient care process, but in which the technical/physiological domain remains the core work and the medical expert manages the overall care process. Nurses acknowledge the difference in occupational focus, but increas-ingly seek to claim a degree of shared expertise in the technical domain, and also question whether this domain has primacy over other personal and social aspects of the care process. They are more likely to aspire to a 'different but equal' model of teamwork.

These responses illustrate that what is at issue is a moral as well as a technical division of labour (see also Chapter 5, this volume). Doctors' and nurses' perceptions of their technical roles are embedded in understandings about the proper form of social relations and the relative value of different aspects of the work. These attributions of value are communicated in indirect ways but are central to the competing discourses touched upon earlier, which on the one hand frame the technical/physiological dimension as core medical work, and on the other hand sketch out a more diffuse vision of holistic, whole-person care. Each in turn implies a different organisation of work in terms of degrees of role specialisation and arrangements for managing the team. These understandings shape doctors' and nurses' conceptualisations of teams and teamwork.

Many of our interviews unfold according to a particular dynamic which illustrates this point. They follow a pattern whereby respondents start out by offering an endorsement for an idealised version of teamwork, based on greater equality and mutual dialogue, which then seems to be partially undercut as the respondent is probed about the detail of what is involved. It is at this point that doctors' and nurses' accounts, that initially portray teamwork as a good thing, diverge to reveal the differences sketched out in previous sections, and where both start to make references to the continuing significance of hierarchy. At face value this process resembles the shift from 'public' to 'private' accounts described by Cornwall (1984). Public accounts are sets of meanings that reaffirm an ideology or moral order that is taken to be acceptable to the audience involved; they are constructed to accord with approved social or organisational norms and not cause offense. Private accounts on the other hand are derived from experience or personal opinion, and may challenge the approved version of how things are. Cornwell shows how over a series of interviews, and especially as questioning moves from the general to the realm of personal experience, respondents start to contradict or qualify earlier public accounts to reveal a 'darker' side of things. The distinction has been criticised for its tendency towards oversimplification (Frankenberg 1986) and confusion over the criteria for separating the public from the private (Radley and Billig 1996).

However, there was a parallel process in our study by which initial accounts emphasising equality within teams were partially contradicted as the interview progressed by references to hierarchy and the role of doctors as team leaders. As they were required to offer more detail on the reality of teamwork in practice, our respondents were forced to move beyond generalisations to construct accounts of teamwork, which meshed more closely with the everyday realities of their work. In describing what teamwork meant, they also needed to make reference to other components of the value systems of medicine and nursing, which remained important to their everyday practice. In our view these are not so much 'private' accounts, in the sense of deeper personal meanings that respondents wish to keep hidden, as situated constructions of teamwork, in which the 'ideal' must necessarily be elaborated in the light of the respondent's pragmatic understandings of the work. As respondents talked about what teamwork would mean for everyday work, some of the reality of mundane working relationships seeped into their accounts.

As mentioned above, these tensions in respondents' accounts often became visible when they referred to leadership roles. Several nurses, although presenting teamwork as a source of greater equality, acknowledged that it was the doctors who would 'manage' the team.

> I suppose [the doctor is] a manager of the individual's physiological care and obviously social and psychological care as well. But we work on it as a team, even though they may have the more academic background in relation to the individual's physiological state. It's important that you work as a team and they count you as an equal or somebody who can carry out the care. (Staff nurse)

It was also recognised that consultants might be less willing than junior hospital doctors to operate as team players:

> I think it's much more of a team these days, they [doctors] are just another part of the team and you are not afraid to speak to them or to put your point of view forward, not to doctors. Consultants maybe, some consultants are a bit aloof to nursing staff unless you have a navy dress and then they'll speak to you. (Staff nurse)

A number of medical respondents, who voiced support for teamwork, also expressed the view that not all team members were created equal. One senior house officer stated early in his interview that: 'Doctors do regard nurses as part of the team care and not just as people we ask to do things'. But later he explained that just as senior medical colleagues had more influence than junior ones, so nurses had less influence than doctors:

> If you are functioning as a team [...] if you are three doctors on a ward round and you are the most junior, and you differ on some point of treatment which the senior is deciding about, you might make your opinion known but in the end you might realise that the responsibility lies with the senior consultant. So it has to be his decision on what is going to happen. The same thing applies for the nurse/doctor relationship.

The comments of many doctors reflected the 'we decide, you carry it out' division of labour in healthcare described by Cott (1998). These doctors saw the nurse's role as limited to carrying out tasks within the plan devised by the doctor.

> And to translate, I won't say our instructions, but whatever things we want provide for the patient in the way of medication or care, it is very vital that you have a good nurse to do that. Because you can write the drug charts, you can ask for things to be done but if there isn't anybody able or willing to do those. It is also an instrument of our care. Nurse/doctor: I think it's part of a team, it's the most vital role they could play. It's two tyres on a bike. If one of the tyres is not doing well patient care suffers. (Senior house officer)

> As a registrar the nurses are my ears and my eyes. (Registrar)

Some were prepared to go a little further to admit a measure of shared decision making, but only in areas where this was not seen to threaten their 'core' medical expertise. The doctors made strong claims to the leadership role. In the words of one medical respondent, the doctor was seen as the 'inevitable and most appropriate leader of teamwork'. Two main justifications for this were offered, based on differential training and the doctor's legal responsibility for patient care.

> Diagnosing patient's illness would not be appropriate for nurses to do, not because they are a different class or anything like that, but just because their training is orientated differently. Treating patients is not the nurse's role in my opinion. By treating I mean managing or making plans for management. Once a plan for management has been made by somebody who has been trained to make a plan for management, then the best way of implementing the plan is something that is decided then, and the nitty gritty of implementing the plan can be to some extent taken over by the nurses. (Registrar)

> There are a lot of things, about which nurses might make their feelings known, which is fine. It is appreciated. But in the end the decision has

to lie with somebody who has to carry responsibility for the patient. So I don't think it is fair on her part to make suggestions without accepting responsibility. Unless they are happy to accept more responsibility for the ultimate care of the patient I think they will always have to accept that their role is limited to a certain extent. (Senior house officer)

Many of the doctors' comments reflected a strong claim of personal responsibility for patients, and a feeling that in the event of an untoward occurrence it will be the doctor who is held to account. This mindset was reflected in the much-used phrase, 'my patient'.

Our sense is that many nurses at the present time perceive these to be powerful arguments. However, it is not clear that they will have the same strength in the future. The increased provision of advanced nurse training programmes means that many nurses will be able to claim training in these areas, and the rise of the doctrine of vicarious liability in negligence cases means that it is increasingly the organisation rather than the individual doctor who is held responsible in the strict legal sense.

Conclusion

While both doctors and nurses suggested that teamwork is valuable and was being implemented in a range of hospital contexts, most recognised the continuing power of medical hierarchies and the limits of nursing influence in core areas of medical work. Generally, nurses volunteered more optimistic and unqualified views of the extent of joint decision making, while doctors, although supporting the notion of teamwork, felt that it might not apply when diagnosis and the planning of treatments were involved. We are not suggesting that our respondents' statements of support for teamwork should be dismissed as mere rhetoric. However, our findings may support Dingwall's (1980) argument that talking about teamwork is largely a way of making certain sorts of occupational claims rather than a way of concerting action. Doctors' and nurses' constructions of teamwork project their existing values and preoccupations into the new team arena, and map out a vision of that arena which preserves aspects of their existing professional projects. From a slightly different perspective, Campbell-Heider and Pollock (1987: 421) argue that, although both medical and nursing personnel advocate team approaches to patient care, the two professions do so 'for different and possibly incommensurable reasons'.

For the doctors, there is a need to be seen to be politically correct and express support for collegiality and teamwork. However, most doctors' constructions of teamwork implicitly support traditional hierarchies. When they talk of teamwork in the context of everyday ward work, they refer to a team made up of the leader and the led, with the doctor cast in the leadership role. Doctors are most at ease with formal multi-disciplinary teams when their remit is limited to areas of social or organisational decision making that are seen as peripheral to core medical decisions. It might even be argued that their support for such teams amounts to an attempt to mark out an arena for nurse decision-making at the periphery that leaves medicine's 'core' territory intact.

For the nurses, constructing the 'team' as a collegiate affair fits well with nursing's professionalising project. Although nursing influence is confined mainly to peripheral areas of medical decision making, nurses can point to a domain of nursing knowledge that informs at least some decisions. Nurses' inclusion in teams enhances their problem-solving skills and gives improved access to professional networks, which may augment their informal influence. Although doctors do not see formally-constituted multi-disciplinary teams as powerful bodies, they provide a model of teamwork characterised by de-centralised authority and flexible leadership that may in future become more influential (Tempkin-Greener 1983). This is in tune with developments such as 'primary nursing', which may be seen as part of a common drive to create expanded opportunities for autonomous professional practice.

Yet, both positions seem likely to be unsustainable. Nurses have gained a measure of equality in relation to decision making about the social, but doctors are able to construct the work in ways that marginalise the importance of the social in the overall delivery of care. Doctors seek to maintain hierarchies, albeit perhaps in partially-disguised form, but then fail to make full use of human resources in an overstretched health service, and risk being seen as a source of inter-professional friction by overseeing authorities increasingly preoccupied with the problem of clinical governance. In the post-Bristol Royal Infirmary Inquiry NHS, few will wish to be seen as advocates for the dysfunctional, doctor-led teams that attracted such strong criticism in the Inquiry Report. Larson (1999: 43) has stated that: 'If there is an underlying mismatch between the fundamental beliefs of physicians and nurses about the value of collaboration, it will be extremely difficult for them to work together or even side by side'. Our study suggests that this is a problem that will surface again and again as the 'team' concept is rolled out across the NHS.

4 'Routine' and 'emergency' in the PACU: the shifting contexts of nurse–doctor interaction

Morag Prowse and Davina Allen

Introduction

In this chapter we examine nurses' accounts of their interactions with doctors in the post-anaesthesia care unit (PACU). The nurses' descriptions of their working relationships indicate that they employ a range of strategies in negotiating care with medical staff. On the one hand, they point to interactional styles redolent of Stein's (1967) doctor–nurse game; in as much as they preserve the appearance of an asymmetrical power relationship between the two professions. On the other hand, their accounts of emergency situations describe a rather different form of interaction, characterised by increased assertiveness and the adoption of a more overtly directive role for nurses. Drawing on an emergent body of social sciences literature that has started to map the highly situated patterning of doctor–nurse relations, we utilise the nurses' accounts to argue that the importance of professional identities appears to vary according to the context. In the PACU environment medical and nursing tasks overlap and doctors and nurses share a body of knowledge. Although they explicitly recognise their own clinical expertise, the nurses' accounts indicate that during routine work situations they were oriented to the differential power relationships between the two occupational groups and that they adopted interactional styles that displayed respect for doctors' 'professional turf'. This they believed to be necessary to ensure good interpersonal relationships. In the nurses' descriptions of emergency situations when a life might be at stake, however, the occupational statuses of medical and nursing staff appeared to be less important: in these instances the nurses describe interactional styles which were more assertive. In both types of narrative the nurses account for their actions in terms of the benefits for patient outcomes.

Background

The characteristics of the nurse–doctor relationship have fascinated observers for many years. This is reflected in media portrayals of doctors and nurses at work and the plethora of hospital romances in which the doctor and the nurse are the main protagonists. Widely regarded as the pivotal relationship in the delivery of healthcare, it has also received sustained scrutiny by the academic community. Authors from various analytic perspectives (e.g. Stein 1967; Dingwall 1977; Gamarnikow 1978; Keddy et al. 1986; Hughes 1988; Stein et al. 1990; Mackay 1993; Walby and Greenwell et al. 1994; Porter 1995; Svensson 1996; Allen 1997; Wicks 1998) have described nurse–doctor interactions in healthcare contexts. Taken together, this body of work has highlighted the complexity of the nurse–doctor relationship which, at one level is characterised by medical dominance (Freidson 1970b) and a gendered division of labour in which nurses care and doctors cure (Gamarnikow 1978) and yet, at another, is located in a changing healthcare scene which produces a blurring of the caring and curing functions and circumstances in which experienced nurses are frequently more knowledgeable than their medical colleagues (Hughes 1988; Allen 1997, see also Chapters 2 and 3, this volume).

Interpreting the literature in this area is a difficult task. It spans a 30-year period during which time important macrosociological changes have occurred affecting medical–nursing relations. Second wave feminism has led to an increased awareness of the politics of gender and changed the expectations and interactional styles of some women. Nursing has been engaged in a 'professional project' (Larson 1977) whereby occupational leaders have sought to assert nurses' identity as autonomous professionals with parity of status with doctors. Furthermore, economic and technological developments have seen an increased blurring of the tasks undertaken by medical and nursing staff, with the development of nurse practitioner roles and the expansion of nursing jurisdiction into areas of work previously the exclusive jurisdiction of medicine. At the same time, social scientific scholarship has itself developed, resulting in more sophisticated frameworks for understanding patterns of social interaction.

Possibly taking the lead from Freidson's (1970b) writings on medical dominance, for many years social scientists tended to view nurse–doctor relations in terms of a straightforward subordination of nursing to medical staff. Scholars pointed to the control the medical profession exerted over nursing's knowledge base and the extent to which, in their daily practice, nurses worked under medical direction. Moreover, an implicit assumption in many of these early studies was the existence of a clear jurisdictional boundary between medical and nursing work. In other words, doctors were assumed to cure and the nursing role restricted to caring functions. As scholarship in this area has advanced, however, it has become apparent that the doctor–nurse relationship is not as straightforward as early models had implied.

Examining nurse–physician interaction in a psychiatric setting, Rushing (1965) suggested that although nurses exhibited deferential styles of interaction, this could be interpreted as an attempt to gain overall influence over the course of treatment rather than an unproblematic display of occupational subordination. According to Rushing, although the doctor supposedly has superior knowledge, a situation may often arise when the nurse, because of their proximity to the patient, may feel they know more than the doctor does. Rushing argues that because of the status differential between nursing and medicine, if the nurse questioned the doctor s/he risked damaging the doctor–nurse relationship. According to Rushing, the nurses' 'power strategies ... are influence at the price of deference: she (sic) attempts to 'exchange' her deference behaviour for a change in the doctors' treatment plan' (Rushing 1965: 372).

It is, however, Stein's (1967) account of the 'doctor–nurse game' that has been the most influential qualification of the traditional model of medical dominance (Hughes 1988). At the time that it was written, Stein's game metaphor captured the imagination of both social theorists and academic nurses and even today continues to be regularly cited in the literature. Stein highlighted the ways that nurses 'blurred' occupational boundaries, when they used their knowledge and experience to influence patient care, while still maintaining a show of deference to the doctors. In this way nurses were able to communicate recommendations which, in retrospect, appear to have been initiated by the doctor. Although Stein (1967) provides no empirical evidence to support his insights, the paper challenged previously accepted ideas about the relationships between nursing and medicine. More recent work, however, indicate that nurses are less concerned with preserving appearances of medical dominance and will interact with their medical colleagues in a direct way (Hughes 1988; Stein *et al.* 1990; Porter 1995; Allen 1997; see also Chapter 2, this volume).

Hughes's (1988) account of expertise in a casualty department revealed nurses to be less concerned with a 'show of subservience' than the game metaphor implies. In analysing his data, Hughes notes that in almost all cases that involved a breakdown of traditional deference, the doctors involved were juniors, relatively inexperienced and came from overseas. He explains his findings partly in terms of the differential local knowledge of the doctors and nurses in this study and, partly in terms of the dilemmas and contradictions in status involved in the relations between young, inexperienced, overseas casualty officers and mature, indigenous nurses.

Reviewing the literature, Porter (1991) identifies four ideal types of nurse–doctor interaction: unproblematic subordination, informal covert decision making (Stein 1967), informal overt decision making (Hughes 1988) and formal overt decision making (the 'nursing process'). He examines these ideal types in relation to empirical evidence collected through participant observation in an intensive care unit and a general medical ward. Porter argues that closer inspection suggest that these models of nurse–doctor interaction may be more complex than has previously been assumed. For example, he argues that what appears to be a case of unproblematic subordination reveals a more subtle form of interaction: doctors frequently offered nurses explanations and justification for their decisions. Moreover, greater scope for nursing input is provided for than is allowed by the traditional model. *Apropos* Stein's 'doctor–nurse game', Porter points out that although the model recognises that the explicit identification of a problem carries with it an implicit suggestion as to its solution, it fails to acknowledge that often the possible solutions are so well understood by doctors and nurses that there is little extra information to be gained by the nurse in spelling out the suggestion.

As well as indicating scholarly progress, the findings of Hughes and Porter may also reflect changing social attitudes towards gender relations that have taken place since Stein's work was first published. Writing in 1990, Stein and colleagues remark on the changes that have occurred in the nurse–doctor game since the original paper in the 1960s. These authors maintain that in many places the nurse–doctor game is still alive and well but they believe that the forces in play forecast change. The factors that Stein *et al.* (1990) point to, include: the declining public esteem for the doctor, the increase in female physicians, the decline of the nurses' handmaiden image and the rise of professional consciousness. These authors see the move towards increased autonomy for nurses as a result of the women's movement. Stein and associates argue that increasingly nurses feel free to confront and even challenge physicians on issues of patient care.

At the macro-sociological level, then, the passage of time clearly impacts upon professional relationships and the literature indicates movement towards mixed patterns of nurse–doctor interaction. If patterns of nurse–doctor interaction are more variable than hitherto recognised, then the question arises as to what factors affect the form that it takes in a given clinical context. There are some clues in the literature in relation to this. We saw, in Hughes's (1988) work for example, how other aspects of social status – such as ethnicity – serve to mediate professional boundaries. Another factor, which is clearly significant in the case of doctors and nurses, is gender. Tellis-Nayak and Tellis-Nayak (1984) argue that female nurses perceive that the patronising attitude of male physicians loses its edge when it is a male nurse in question. These authors conclude that the gender and race components of interactional behaviour in the wider culture carries over and colours professional interactions.

[T]he norms of inequality of the sexes and of the inequality of the professional status conspire in a hospital setting and consolidate the subordinate position of the nurse in her social conversation with the physician. (Tellis-Nayak and Tellis-Nayak 1984: 1068)

Observational studies suggest that doctor–nurse relations may be also mediated by context (Coser 1962; Rosengren and Devault 1963; Wessen 1958; Millman 1976; Mumford 1970). Relations between doctors and nurses vary according to the type of hospital (Mumford 1970) or the ward structure (Coser 1962). In their analysis of time and space in an obstetric hospital, Rosengren and Devault (1963) observed differential behaviour of the nurses towards doctors, interns and medical students according to place. Key to this was whether the patient was present and could overhear what was being said. Within earshot of patients, nurses exhibited more respect. In the delivery room with the patients under anaesthesia, the demeanour of the nurses towards the younger interns frequently changed to giving orders and calling them by their last name only. Similar observations were made by Wilson (1958) in the operating theatre. What these studies point to is that one element of nurse–doctor interaction is its orientation to enacting a particular kind of relationship for the benefit of patients. In this way patient confidence is maintained and the appearance of consensus in the healthcare team is preserved.

Shifting contexts of nurse–doctor interaction in the PACU

Although they do not explicitly present themselves in these terms, these studies indicate that the nurse–doctor boundary is both a division of labour and a social relationship and that each of these elements are subject to change, both historically and in response to a given social context. This brings to mind Hughes's (1984) classic distinction between the technical and the moral division of labour. In his writings on the world of work and occupations Hughes underlined the importance of distinguishing the work, that is, the tasks to be accomplished, from the worker. He recognised that the division of labour was forever changing in response to macro-sociological and micro-sociological factors, and he drew attention to the processes through which types of work and 'bundles of tasks' could be shifted from one occupational group to another in response to such influences. Hughes was interested in the general features of work and workers of all kinds, but he recognised that certain kinds of work and different types of worker were accorded more or less social esteem in a given society. In other words, both work and workers had differential status or moral value. One of the ways an occupation could attempt to increase its status was by taking on work that was accorded high social value.

Although Hughes used the concept of 'the division of labour' in his writings, he was never entirely at ease with it. For him it connoted divisions and separations, whereas he saw the world of work as an intricate system. According to Hughes it was impossible to understand the work of an individual without giving due consideration to the work of those with whom they interact within the workplace. It is at the level of face-to-face interaction that occupational statuses are accomplished and the allocation of work takes place.

Following on from Hughes and studies of nurse–doctor relations we explore patterns of nurse–doctor interaction in the PACU. We draw on interviews with nurses working in PACU which indicate that the definition of a situation as routine or emergency shapes both the allocation of work and the attention participants appear to place on occupational status differences. The nurses' descriptions of their work in PACU indicate that they employ a range of interaction styles with doctors that appear to be adapted to the context in order to optimise particular patient outcomes. Although distinctive features of this clinical setting led to a fluid division of tasks between medical and nursing staff, in their routine interactions with doctors, nurses demonstrated a respect for their medical colleagues' professional turf and their descriptions of their interactions revealed many features of Stein's game model. However, when nurses formulated the patient's condition as constituting an emergency then their accounts indicated that occupational boundaries were more willingly crossed and a more directive interactional style was described.

The study

The paper draws on data arising from a wider study which sought to describe the ways that experienced nurses used 'effective' knowledge, derived in part from the biosciences, in post-anaesthesia nursing practice to achieve intended patient outcomes (Prowse and Lyne 2000a,b). The study utilised narrative data, generated through in-depth interviews with 32 experienced post-anaesthesia nurses. This clinical setting was selected because it was an unexamined area of nursing practice and the researcher (MP) has specialist skill and knowledge which helped in gaining entry to the field, securing the co-operation of participants and interpreting clinically-based data. As the development of nursing knowledge and experience were focal points of the study, participants were purposively selected, first, on the basis of their willingness to take part and, second, so as to include a continuum of experience. In-depth interviews were carried out in two phases over a year; each tape-recorded, transcribed verbatim and supplemented by field notes representing the researcher's thoughts and observations about the interview process. The nurses were asked to illustrate their experiences of post-anaesthesia nursing practice by describing incidents where their knowledge or experience had influenced a patient outcome. Although the nurses were not specifically asked about patterns of nurse–doctor interaction, these featured in all the accounts. Clearly, there are methodological issues in extrapolating from interview accounts to everyday practice and the study of social interactions is best undertaken using ethnographic field methods (Silverman 1993). However, what the nurses' accounts do indicate is something of the 'scene' in the day-to-day work of the nurses in the PACU and provide some clues as to the possible mediating factors which shape social interaction in healthcare settings. They also communicate moral realities, revealing the shared interpretative resources through which nurses construct their occupational role and position themselves in relation to members of other occupational groups (Allen 2001b).

Inter-professional working in PACU

Fluid boundaries and shared knowledge

Patient care in the PACU is delivered in a multi-disciplinary context where medical, nursing and other occupational boundaries intersect in the delivery of care. Some of these boundaries are legal ones that cannot be transgressed, while others are more flexible and fluid and can be modified depending on the circumstances. Some examples of legal professional boundaries in the PACU, in the UK, are specialised activities such as tracheal intubation of patients and the administration of general anaesthesia. Medical practitioners who have undergone specialist education in anaesthesia can only carry out these tasks. Thus, this is a legally defined boundary between the role of the PACU nurse and the role of an anaesthetist which the staff would not transgress.

Other task areas have more fluid boundaries although, technically, law too circumscribes them. One example is the prescription and consequent administration of oxygen and intravenous fluids in the PACU. Legally, doctors should prescribe both, in writing, before either is administered. In day-to-day working practice, however, this is not adhered to and experienced staff will normally administer oxygen or fluids in emergency situations to ensure that the patient's situation is not compromised by delay (see also Chapter 2, this volume). The data from our study suggest that the nurses perceived a difference between some legally defined boundaries and others in terms of the skill and knowledge required to undertake these roles safely. Intubation and administration of anaesthesia are complex skills requiring advanced knowledge and expertise, whereas administration of oxygen and fluids to stabilise a patient until medical advice is sought is within the scope and remit of a registered nurse. The different roles carried out by medical and nursing staff in the PACU are reflected in the stages of the patient's progression through the operating theatre. At some points on this journey, medical staff are in constant attendance while at others, there is no immediately available doctor. The patient arrives at the operating theatre complex awake and is rendered unconscious in the anaesthetic room. From here, the unconscious patient enters the operating theatre and then makes the journey back to consciousness in the post-anaesthesia care unit. Thus, the patient follows a temporal–spatial 'trajectory' through the various 'workshops' (Strauss *et al.* 1985) which comprise the operating theatre world. The timing and flow of work means that an anaesthetist is either in the operating theatre, in the anaesthetic room, in the PACU or in transit between these areas. Clearly, s/he cannot be in all three places at once and this 'temporal–spatial' feature creates a situation where nurses develop skills and competence in order to ensure continuity of patient care in the absence of the anaesthetist.

Allen (1997) has shown how the 'temporal–spatial' organisation of ward work can lead to the routine blurring of medical and nursing tasks (see also Chapter 2, this volume). Similarly, in the PACU, although certain interventions are professionally differentiated – for example, prescribing, tracheal intubation and insertion of central lines are restricted to anaesthetists – patient care centres on 'interventions' which are aimed at restoring physiological stability with the consequence that the boundary between medical work and nursing work is particularly 'fluid'. Rather than being assigned along conventional lines of occupational delineation, many interventions in the PACU are allocated according to level of expertise, competence and confidence.

Examples of interventions in the PACU are 'maintaining the airway', 'achieving optimum analgesia', 'stabilising blood pressure' and 'ensuring adequate oxygenation'. They cannot be usefully classified as 'medical' or 'nursing', because either doctors or nurses carry them out in the same way. In this respect, PACU nursing has much in common with intensive and critical care nursing: compared to other healthcare settings there is far less demarcation between 'tasks' that people undertake and their professional role.

Negotiation space(s)

Svensson (1996) introduced the concept of 'negotiation space' into the literature on nurse–doctor relations in his study of Swedish nursing. Drawing on the negotiated order perspective

(Strauss *et al.* 1963, 1985), he argues that in recent years changes in the healthcare context have created 'space' for nurses to directly influence patient care decisions and augment their influence *vis-à-vis* the medical profession. For example, he points to the increased prevalence of chronic illness that has introduced a social dimension into healthcare. According to Svensson, nurses are powerfully placed to contribute to patient management, given the centrality of 'the social' to holistic care (see also Chapter 3, this volume). There were various features of the PACU that created negotiation-space for nursing staff.

Although compared to nurses, medical staff are typically educated to a higher level in the biological sciences, the social organisation of work in PACU settings leads to a situation where nurses have greater experience which gives them a clinical 'feel' that is not shared by their medical colleagues. Nurses are permanent staff members whereas, in a given locale, doctors rotate around clinical areas. Doctors also work an 'on call' pattern where they are responsible for large areas whereas nurses work prescribed shifts in specific domains. As a number of authors have noted, the relative transience and permanence of doctors and nurses can influence nurse–doctor relations in important ways (Hughes 1988; Walby and Greenwell *et al.* 1994; Porter 1995; Allen 1997). In the PACU the nursing staff were the PACU 'natives' in contrast to the transient 'tourist' status of junior doctors. These features created a situation where new doctors found themselves in unfamiliar work areas on a regular basis.

Experienced PACU nurses demonstrated a particular kind of knowledge which mediated the medical–nursing boundary in the PACU. This was defined in the study as 'effective knowledge' because it was developed in the clinical setting and was influential in activating intended patient outcomes. Effective knowledge is a descriptor, adapted from empirical educational research of the kind of knowledge developed from problem solving in everyday life situations (e.g. Lave 1988a,b; Brown *et al.* 1989). In a similar way to Benner's (1984) expert nurses, the PACU practitioners' accounts revealed extensive knowledge of typical patient problems and their associated interventions.

PACU is a critical care area and an example of a 'turbulent' (Melia 1979) work context. Because of the relative physiological instability of the perioperative patient, and the intermittent 'flow' of patients, 'chaos' and unpredictable events punctuate periods of predictable and routine work. A defining feature of PACU work is therefore its 'fast time frame'. What this means is that when a situation of physiological instability occurs, there are minutes to recognise the problem and initiate the appropriate interventions. The PACU nurses need a high level of skill in order to ensure patient safety because the interventions are urgent and medical assistance may be some distance and time away.

Two types of clinical event can be categorised: routine and emergency. In routine clinical situations, the changes in the patient's physiological parameters were anticipated and the experienced nurses dealt with these everyday situations by following established protocols and procedures. An example of a routine change in a post anaesthesia patient's physiological status is the transient drop in blood pressure and slowing of respiratory rate which often follows the administration of drugs such as Morphine for post-operative pain. When patients in ward situations develop low blood pressure and slowing of respiratory rate, these clinical changes are likely to be interpreted by nurses as constituting an emergency because of the potential for serious consequences if uncorrected. In the PACU, however, these physiological variations are an everyday occurrence. Moreover, patients are monitored continuously, and minute by minute physiological variations allow immediate action to be taken to correct any problems. An emergency in the PACU was a situation of rapid, and usually accelerating, physiological change that was unexpected and would result in the death of the patient if not immediately corrected. Hypoxia is one example where physiological changes, indicated by readings on a pulse oximeter, indicate that the level of oxygen available to the patient is within a 'danger zone' which leaves around three minutes to take preventative action. The experienced PACU nurses understood the context of these physiological changes and the immediacy of the particular time frame in ways which less experienced doctors sometimes failed to appreciate. Situations of rapid physiological change and the immediacy of the time frame created by the patient's potential deterioration, placed inexperienced doctors in a position of uncertainty. In this way, a 'negotiation space' (Svensson 1996) was created. When doctors failed to identify these particular problems, and make the correct decision about managing those problems in the relevant time frame, nurses intervened. Nevertheless, although routine PACU work led nurses to cross the medical–nursing boundary, their accounts of such incidents reveal a careful management of the situation in which elements of the nurse–doctor game figure prominently. This indicates that although nurses were prepared to move outside of their own task area, they were nevertheless oriented to doctors' occupational status as the expert in a given domain of work. However, in situations defined by nurses as an emergency, their descriptions suggest that the doctor's occupational status was less important. Nurses describe interactional styles that were more challenging and directive. These data suggest that nurses may purposefully modify their interactions with doctors according to the context in order to achieve patient outcomes.

Interactional styles and negotiation space

'Routine' interactions

Although the nurses' descriptions revealed the existence of effective knowledge derived from their experience working in PACU, they were also clearly oriented to the existence of an occupational boundary between nursing and medical staff. In the following extracts, for example, the nurses talk about the existence of boundaries which cannot be transgressed and the discomfiture experienced if they feel that they have 'overstepped the mark' in making suggestions about clinical treatments to medical staff.

Extract 1

MP: Does everyone have a style for working in PACU?

26: Everybody has a different style but we all try to maintain the same standards, we all know the standards and the protocols, and nobody oversteps the boundary, but certain people work at different levels, even then. *But we all know there are boundaries that you cannot step over.*

(Participant 26 – 8 years PACU experience – our emphasis)

In this extract the nurse makes a distinction between those tasks routinely carried out by nurses and those that can be carried out only by anaesthetists in the PACU. What she appears to point to is that even in an occupational setting such as the PACU in which there is a fluidity of occupational boundaries because knowledge and skill overlap, staff still recognise specific zones of responsibility. Often, these task differentials relate more to occupational restrictions than knowledge and skill. For example, only anaesthetists in the UK carry out the intubation of patients but in Europe and North America it is a routine role for nurse anaesthetists. The nurse describes how it is boundaries, such as this, that she would not step over. The next extract shows a similar perception of boundaries between the nurse's role and the anaesthetist's role but in this extract, the nurse is prepared to negotiate on the patient's behalf.

Extract 2

MP: Are there any decisions in PACU on a day-to-day basis that are more difficult than others to make?

19: I think when you feel like you've come to the end of the line in terms of analgesia for instance, with the patient. And you've been back to the anaesthetist and the anaesthetist says 'Well, I don't think it's appropriate to give any more analgesia for this patient.' And you feel maybe that they're right, that it isn't appropriate, but the patient still feels that they should have more, or that you feel that in that case they do need more analgesia, so that situation of trying to manage, then of *stepping over that line again*, if you like, saying 'Well actually I feel like this patient does need more' [...] It makes me *uncomfortable* dealing with the anaesthetist, because even though I'm confident of my assessment, that anaesthetist is not always going to agree, and you try, *there is only so far you can push it*, in that situation.

MP: And ultimately the decision about prescribing the drugs is actually theirs isn't it?

19: Yes. And you have to recognise that. And it can leave you feeling frustrated. And I'm sure it must leave some of the anaesthetists feeling that you have *over-stepped the mark, if you like*.

(Participant 19 – female with 7 years PACU experience and specialist education – our emphasis)

This account indicates that the nurse's actions are restrained by her perception of a boundary between herself, dealing with the patient in pain, and the anaesthetist who is responsible for prescribing the analgesia. She expresses her concern about 'stepping over that line' when she asks for further analgesia and describes how the anaesthetist may not agree with her assessment. Although she describes her confidence in these situations, she perceives the doctor as the ultimate decision-maker because s/he has prescribing power. This extract has a number of interesting features. First, together with extract 1, the nurses' description indicates that the PACU staff seems to distinguish between certain areas of knowledge that can be shared and those that cannot. Professional regulatory and legal frameworks are obviously important – in this extract the incident centres on the doctor's legal responsibility for prescribing medications – and although they may not shape the medical–nursing boundary in a deterministic way (see also Chapter 2, this volume) they are clearly influential in shaping the negotiation of occupational boundaries. As this nurse observes, 'there is only so far you can push it'. Second, the nurses' account is clearly framed in terms of her responsibilities for the patient. Her description positions her as the patient's advocate. She knows the patient has been given as much analgesia as is considered clinically appropriate, but she accepts that the patient still wants more and is therefore prepared to 'push' the nursing–medical boundary in the patient's interests. This framing of the situation in terms of working for the patient was a feature of many of the nurses' accounts, irrespective of whether the narrative described an emergency or a routine incident and, it is an issue to which we will return.

Our data indicate that one way in which nurses managed the sensitivity of the medical–nursing boundary was through the adoption of the kinds of indirect interactional styles described by Stein. For example, they talked in terms of 'prompting' and 'guiding' medical staff in order to alert them to salient features of the patient's condition. There are clear parallels here with Hughes's (1988) work in which he highlights how nurses used 'subtle cues' to steer doctors toward a particular course of action. In the following extract, an experienced PACU nurse describes how she uses 'prompts' in order to get an inexperienced doctor to act in a situation that she considered demanded a response.

Extract 3

20: We get quite a lot [of incidents] where, especially at the moment, we've got a lot of junior doctors; you're feeling that you've got to *prompt* them totally. It's just like, the other day we had a patient, who it was very obvious that he was either toxic or hypoxic. Retaining CO_2 or something, and it was an inexperienced anaesthetist, and you just couldn't get her to do anything. I mean, in the end she went, off her own back, and got the senior doctor down, and then it was arterial lines, but we were trying to *prompt* her, saying, 'Do you want this, do you want that?' And she just wasn't, she was like, 'No, no, we'll just wait and see how it goes.'

(Participant 20 – female with 8 years PACU experience and specialist education – our emphasis)

In this extract the nurse recounts how she recognises the need for a clinical intervention and attempts to get the junior doctor to act. Notice how the account is again constructed around the nurses' concern for the patient's welfare. The nurse begins by describing how she made a differential diagnosis, that is, identified more than one possible cause of the patient's problem, in the utterance 'he was either toxic, hypoxic or retaining CO_2'. She tries to effect a clinical intervention by prompting the junior doctor with the questions: 'Do you want this? Do you want that?' Although the junior doctor did not respond directly to the nurses' cues, her interactional style appeared to have effected involvement of the senior doctor who intervened to stabilise the patient's condition. The narrative suggests an interactional encounter in which, the 'social order' of doctors as decision makers in bio-physiological matters was maintained, and the patient outcome achieved, without overt inter-professional conflict.

Extract 4 is another example of an indirect interactional strategy in which the nurse describes how she attempted to persuade a doctor to prescribe medication in a form which was specific to the PACU setting and quite different from its conventional usage.

Extract 4

MP: Can you think of any situation where your knowledge or experience made a difference to a patient outcome?

22: Something does spring to mind as well: I'm quite interested in the post-anaesthetic shivering, which occurs quite a lot, although not as much as it used to. We had a patient, and we had a new intake of anaesthetists and I had a patient shivering that wasn't settling. I suggested to the anaesthetist, I said to her, 'What do you think about Pethidine?' And she said, 'I don't know anything about it.' I said, 'Well, actually it does work but there's an anaesthetist over there, why don't you just ask him and maybe he will clarify it for you.' So she came back and she said, 'Yes, I'll have twenty-five milligrams of Pethidine.' So she [the anaesthetist] learned from that as well.

MP: You handled that very diplomatically, because you referred her to another anaesthetist, even though you knew what to do. Was that to save her face?

22: Yes, I think, yes rather than take it from me, I thought, well, actually he just appeared at the right time, so she just had a word with him. And because of that, I actually found some literature written by one of the anaesthetists who had done a paper on post-operative shivering.

(Participant 22 – female with 9 years PACU experience and specialist education – our emphasis)

In this extract, the nurse makes it clear that she is knowledgeable about post-anaesthetic shivering when she asks 'What do you think about Pethidine?' Her knowledge is *effective* knowledge because the normal usage of this particular drug is for analgesia. In the PACU, Pethidine is given in lower dosages as a treatment for post-anaesthesia shivering. The knowledge is therefore specific to this area of practice.

The nurses' account indicates that the anaesthetist in question is part of a new intake, and therefore inexperienced. As such he cannot be expected to possess knowledge specific to the PACU context. Indeed the nurse recounts how he admits that he does not know anything about post-anaesthesia shivering. The nurse describes how she directs the junior anaesthetist to a more senior colleague; her account is oriented to the 'norm' that doctors usually seek advice about prescribing, a medical role, from other doctors. The doctor follows the guidance given and prescribes the drug advised by the nurse. A professional boundary, prescribing, was observed, but purposeful interactions blurred this boundary as the nurse advised the doctor in a sensitive way.

There are clear parallels in the above extracts with features of Stein's doctor–nurse game. In a work environment in which nursing and medical tasks overlap, the nurses' accounts of their interactions with doctors appear to demonstrate a respect for doctors' turf. These data indicate that nurses believed this to be necessary in order to maintain good interprofessional relationships and they couch this in terms of patient outcomes. In the following extract, the nurse describes her understanding about the need to 'maintain good relationships' and the consequences of failure to do so.

Extract 5

MP: Does challenging the doctors sometimes lead to problems in working relationships?

19: There can be a lot of frustration, probably on the anaesthetist's side as well as ours. And it's how you approach the subject of leading them, I think, a lot of the time. If you have the confidence there, not being cocky and saying, 'Well, I know this is better.' Saying, 'What do you think? Do you think this might work?' Leading, diplomatically if you like, because if not then tensions are going to build up and at the end of the day it's that patient that'll suffer, not you. Well, you might, but at the end of the day you'll find the anaesthetist's not coming to you because you're so stroppy with them, and they think that you're too stroppy and they don't want to listen to what you've got to say, then the patient's not going to get what they need.

(Participant 19 – female with 7 years PACU experience and specialist education – our emphasis)

The nurse's account provides insight into her understanding of the reciprocal nature of professional relationships in the PACU. She talks about mutual feelings of discomfort and frustration which may ensue from challenging a doctor and the sanctions that might be applied, if nurses were not diplomatic with the doctors: doctors not 'coming to them' (nurses) and 'not listening to them' (nurses), which could result in patients not getting 'what they needed'. Here then, respecting each other's professional role is described as integral to the achievement of optimum patient outcomes in the PACU.

Whilst nurses orient to traditional role boundaries in their routine interactions with medical staff, our data indicate that in situations defined by the nurse as emergencies, the occupational statuses of doctors and nurses were less important. In these situations the nurses' accounts indicate that they were more challenging.

The 'challenge' of an 'emergency'

Extract 6

MP: Can you think of any incident when your knowledge or experience made a difference to a patient outcome?

10: It comes [the ability to problem solve] with experience. I recognised a patient who collapsed his lung after he'd had a nephrectomy. They [the doctors] couldn't get his saturations up so they pulled out the equipment and were re-intubating and everything else. They hadn't considered a pneumothorax and I said, 'Look, could we get an X-ray?' They said, 'What do you want an X-ray for?' And I said, 'I'm not happy, and the patient is complaining of shoulder tip pain and no pain in the area where he'd had the operation.' His nail beds were really quite blue. His saturations were 96% on 15 litres [of oxygen] so they weren't too bad. That's why they said there were not too worried about him, but I felt there was something wrong. I hadn't actually seen a pneumothorax before. I'd read about it and I'd listened to one of the doctors querying it on another patient, because of the pattern of the patient's breathing. Because of where the incision site was it was easy for them [the surgeons] to slip and go through the pleura. So putting it all together, knowing what the operation was and with the other signs and symptoms.

MP: Did the doctor listen to you?

10: He did. He said 'we'll do a chest X-ray' and it was an enormous pneumothorax taking up most of his right lung, he only had a small part of his right lung, the upper lobe left.

(Participant 10 – female nurse with 6 years PACU nursing experience – our emphasis)

In this extract the nurse describes herself as directly requesting an X-ray, a task normally the preserve of the doctor. The nurse's question 'Look could we get an X-ray?' is indicative of a more directive interactional style, contrasting with the 'guiding' evident in the previous extract in which the nurse asks 'What do you think about Pethidine?' Although there are also features of the doctor–nurse game in this extract, the 'challenge' is revealed in the nurse's response to the doctor's question: 'What do you want an X-ray for?' Her reply presents her 'standing her ground' about the need for the X-ray: 'I'm not happy, and the patient is complaining of shoulder tip pain and no pain in the area where he'd had the operation'. The nurses' account indicates that faced with a situation she defined as an emergency, the occupational status of the doctor *qua* doctor was less consequential for the way in which she interacted with him.

Extract 7 is another account of an emergency situation. Once again the narrative casts the nurse in a more assertive role.

Extract 7

MP: Can you remember any patient care situations where the patient deteriorated and you had to take some action [...].

25: It was quite an elderly man who'd come out of theatre, he'd had a big surgery, oesophageal gastrectomy. He came out mid-afternoon, and he wasn't very well when he came out, he sort of came out a bit [...] semiconscious, as they do. Which was nothing untoward about that, and his chest [...] very barrel-chested and difficulty breathing and COAD [chronic obstructive airways disease], he had an epidural in, chest drain, but he was very responsive. 'Hello, stick your tongue out, do you know where you are?' 'Yes' [...] Within five minutes, now I'd a new nurse who was looking after him and I was sort of hovering, and the anaesthetist was also around as cover for us, looking after another man who wasn't very well. I disappeared for a couple of minutes to do something else and came back and thought, 'Well this man...'. Within five minutes he just wasn't as conscious as he might have been. This is what worried me. And his breathing was really very much more difficult, so the staff nurse – who was new – I could see her going to the anaesthetist and she was looking at this fellow, so I knew she'd picked it up. The anaesthetist came over. 'Oh he's all right. He was like this when he came out' I said 'No he wasn't' 'He was' he said. 'I was here when Dr Adams handed over' I said, 'He was conscious, responsive and now he isn't. And look at his breathing' Pulse, blood pressure, saturations, were all as they were, normal and acceptable. But this anaesthetist he was just, he was young and he was 'Oh he was like that. He's got a bad chest you know, he's ...' 'But I knew, and I said, look this man needs some intervention'. I immediately went, I went round to the head of his bed and I started to maintain his airway, because he was really struggling and his 'sats' were falling, so I put a Waters Circuit on. Meanwhile the anaesthetist just stood there looking. And then said, 'I think you're right actually, Sister I think he does need some help.'

(Participant 25 – female nurse with 10 years PACU experience and specialist education – our emphasis)

This is an example of a routine event becoming an emergency in the PACU. The nurse's account indicates a change in her interactional style, as she perceives the fast time frame and the particular patient context. The extract describes a series of events where the nurse directly challenges the anaesthetist's judgement when an elderly patient's condition deteriorates. Again the narrative is centred on the need to ensure an optimum patient outcome.

The early part of the text outlines how the experienced nurse passively observes the patient's condition. It then moves on to describe how the nurse observes changes in the elderly patient's consciousness and respiratory pattern which she assesses as significant. The nurse intervenes and draws the less experienced anaesthetist's attention to the salient features of this case. According to the nurse, the less experienced doctor has failed to anticipate the imminent hypoxia (hypoxia is a term used to describe a critical shortage of oxygen available to the tissues which, if not immediately corrected, can cause death) that constitutes an emergency and could result in this patient's death. She describes how she gives respiratory assistance as the patient's saturations (the level of oxygen in body tissues) fall and the hypoxia becomes apparent on the monitor. The nurse recounts how she 'put a Waters Circuit on'. This is a form of assisted ventilation and is normally the task of the anaesthetist. On this occasion, however, the nurse transgresses this occupational boundary and initiates this procedure. According to the nurses' narrative, the anaesthetist gradually comes to accept her assessment that this is an emergency and that intervention is required. Unlike some of the other extracts where experienced nurses describe their hesitation because of a perceived boundary, in this situation the nurse is clearly less orientated to the doctor's occupational status. Her account stresses her overriding concern with the patient's interests. The negotiation space of the PACU emergency creates a situation where roles are reversed and the doctor comes close to following the nurse's directions.

Discussion and conclusions

In this paper, we have examined PACU nurses' accounts of their day-to-day interactions with doctors. Their descriptions indicate that the nurses adapted their interactional style according to context. In PACU, negotiation space (Svensson 1996) was created around the fast 'time-frame' of critical incidents, the temporal–spatial features of the work and the relative experience of nurse and doctor. The nurses' accounts describe how they combine their 'effective knowledge' with a range of 'negotiation styles' to achieve patient outcomes. We have suggested that in their routine interactions with medical staff, nurses' reported accounts appeared to display many features of Stein's game model. Their descriptions portray interactional styles oriented to a respect for the doctor's professional jurisdiction and their occupational status. Although situated knowledge and expertise, mediated by features of the clinical setting, placed nurses in situations where they were frequently more knowledgeable than inexperienced medical colleagues, they also recognised the importance of not offending them. By playing the 'game' nurses ensured that the doctors continued to come to them for advice. In their accounts of emergency situations, however, nurses described their interactional styles as more assertive and focused entirely on achieving patient outcomes. Status differences between nurses and doctors are apparently less relevant when staff are faced with a life and death situation.

There are clear links here with the findings of other studies in the literature, which indicate that an individual's social identity varies according to the context. Timmermans (1999), for example, argues that during cardiopulmonary resuscitation (CPR) 'people are reduced to mere bodies, and their dignity is repeatedly violated' (109). Similarly, Lawler (1991) points out, that contrary to nurses' professional rhetoric in which they claim to provide individualised patient care, in order to cross sensitive cultural boundaries it is often necessary for nurses to disengage from the social identities of persons *qua* persons. In the same way, the nurses' accounts indicate that although they were oriented to the occupational identities of doctors during their routine work interactions, this routine interactional frame was temporarily suspended in emergency situations.

Clearly, there are limitations in uncritically treating interview accounts as straightforward indices of actual behaviour (Silverman 1993) but these findings do suggest one way in which nurse–doctor interaction is shaped in daily practice. Furthermore, they communicate the moral realities of an occupational culture. As we have seen, one interesting feature of the data extracts is the way in which nurses construct their accounts around patient, rather than professional, interests. In the stories that they tell and in their accounts of their work 'working for the patient' is a key element in the interpretative repertoire from which nurses rhetorically construct their role and their relationships with other occupational groups (Allen 2001b).

Given the changing boundaries and contexts of contemporary healthcare, it is important to reconsider how patterns of nurse–doctor interaction contribute to effective patient care.

These data indicate that the doctor–nurse game is alive and well in contemporary nursing practice. This will give little comfort to those who argue for nursing's parity of status with medical staff. The PACU nurses interviewed for this study clearly had local knowledge derived from experience and were informed by research, yet they still were cautious about encroaching into medical territory. At the same time, however, their accounts indicate that where deference was highly consequential for patient outcomes, status differences paled in significance.

5 Expanded nursing roles: different occupational perspectives

Davina Allen and David Hughes

Introduction

> [W]e are convinced that more concerted action is needed to encourage changes to skill-mix and more flexible working. Traditional demarcation lines between professional groups and between professional and non-professional groups (e.g. between doctors and nurses or between nurses and health care assistants) are not conducive to delivering high-quality, patient-centred, care. (NHS 2000: 28)

This extract comes from a United Kingdom (UK) government consultation document, which sets out a number of proposals for the future of the National Health Service (NHS) workforce. It proposes a vision of the health services division of labour in which traditional role boundaries are broken down so that staff expertise can be deployed flexibly according to patients' needs. These new arrangements are contrasted with 'traditional demarcation lines', which are presented as 'not conducive to delivering high-quality, patient-centred care.'

Background

Concern with the health services division of labour is by no means new. In fact workforce issues have been a dominant theme in policy making over the last 20 years as the NHS has been restructured many times in response to the breakdown of the post-war consensus over the Welfare State. Widely criticised as inefficient and unresponsive to users, the healthcare sector has experienced a succession of reforms aimed at increasing efficiency, making the services more responsive to users and improving co-ordination. As a labour-intensive industry the health services workforce has always been central to these concerns.

Over the last decade health services staff have witnessed wide ranging changes in the way in which their work is organised and attempts have been made to dismantle traditional lines of demarcation between, for example, doctors and nurses (Allen 1997; Annandale *et al.* 1999) and nurses and health care assistants (HCAs) (Allen 1996, 2000b; Daykin and Clarke 2000). Under the Conservative government market forces provided much of the impetus for many of these changes. The ability to efficiently manage one's own workforce is vitally important in a competitive market (Paton 1993) and in the late 1980s issues of skill mix and workforce re-profiling became key concerns (Paton 1993; Annandale *et al.* 1999). Despite the abolition of the internal market under the 'New Labour' government and a shift from a rhetoric of competition to one of co-operation, workforce issues remain a key concern. It is the exhortation that services should be user-centred that is now the major lever of change. What is interesting about these recent policy developments, however, is the extent to which they have been underpinned by a very particular view of the health services workforce. Berated for their tribalism, turf battles and professional self-interest, health and social services staff have been portrayed as an inherently conservative force. Particular attention has been paid to the need for culture management (Peters and Waterman 1982; Deal and Kennedy 1982) in order to secure organisational change. An implicit objective of the reforms instituted since the 1980s has been to bring managers and professionals into a single framework of accountability (Hughes and Allen 1993a). Under the Conservative government the aim was to create managers out of professionals (Hood 1991) requiring them to be more interested in the costs of services and resource management. The transformation of culture remains a key theme in New Labour policy, but the discourse of consumerism and efficiency has been combined with a rhetoric of quality and partnership.

> The level of change required is significant and is not just about new projects that need funding, or new decision-making structures. It is a key part of the culture change that is taking place in the NHS as

Ministers seek to modernise it to meet patient's demands. (Department
of Health 2000a: 40)

In recent policy documents the health services workforce is
widely portrayed as an obstacle to change in, for example, references to the need to 'break down barriers' and 'work as
teams rather than professional tribes' and in the expressed
concern that 'today's planners do not have to fight yesterday's
battles' (NHS 2000). Yet, workplace based studies on both
sides of the Atlantic undertaken since the 1960s reveal staff to
be extremely flexible in their working practices, prepared to
cross the official boundaries of their role in response to the
demands of the work environment in order to accomplish the
task at hand (Sudnow 1967; Taylor 1970; Roth and Douglas
1983; Hughes 1988; Porter 1991; see also Chapters 2 and 4,
this volume). Indeed, in a recent study of the routine negotiation of roles and responsibilities in the delivery of health and
social services to adults who had sustained a stroke it was
found that it was *only* the willingness of staff to work together
flexibly that made certain complex packages of care possible
(Allen *et al.* 2000). So why is it that ministers persist in por-
traying the health services staff as a conservative force?

One explanation is that it is politically expedient to do so;
blaming NHS staff for the shortcomings of the service deflects
attention away from the thorny question of resource allocation. Some have suggested that NHS governance is an example of a 'wicked issue' (Clarke and Stewart 2000), that is, it is
a 'special class of policy problem; one without an obvious or
established (or even common-sense) solution, defying normal
understanding' (Clarke and Stewart 2000: 377). Seen in this
way, focusing attention on the so-called problem of the NHS
workforce is an attempt to ' "keep on the move", in order to
sustain fluidity and escape responsibilities' (Biggs 2000: 375).

Another possible reason for these apparently contradictory
findings, however, is that they reveal the different ways in
which occupations attempt to shape and control the parameters of their practice. Hughes (1984) considers these processes
in terms of the concepts of 'licence' and 'mandate'. He
employs the notion of licence to denote the activities an occupation is granted to carry out by society and that of mandate
to refer to the claims that are made by an occupation about

the nature of its contribution. The scope of licence and mandate is not fixed; it can expand and contract. Any occupation may attempt to improve its social standing by reconstructing its licence and expanding its mandate. Some occupations have greater power to enlarge their licence and mandate than others do. These processes do not take place in a void of course. As we have outlined in Chapter 1, a number of sociologists have stressed the need to conceptualise the division of labour in society as a social system (Durkheim 1933; Freidson 1976; Hughes 1984; Abbott 1988). Viewed in this way we cannot understand one occupation without reference to those with whom they interact. Changes to the boundaries and work content of one occupation necessarily impact upon others in the system. The system of work is dynamic, moreover; occupational boundaries expand and retreat in response to wider factors such as technological, organisational, social and economic change and against this background occupations vie to elevate their status and improve the conditions of their members (Hughes 1984; Abbott 1988).

Drawing on the work of Hughes (1984, 1958), Abbott (1988) has argued that in order to establish the right to control a particular area of work, occupations have to claim 'jurisdiction'. By jurisdiction he is referring to both the licence and mandate of an occupation. Abbott argues that jurisdictional claims need to be made in public, legal and workplace arenas. In the public arena the professions' self-presentation in, for example, magazines and on the television, aims to portray a particular occupational-image. In America, Abbott claims, it is in the public arena that professionals establish the power that allows them to achieve legal protection. By contrast, in Europe it is the State, which has traditionally been the profession's public, and it is to State officials that professional jurisdictional claims are oriented. Abbott draws attention to the ways in which jurisdictional claims in the public domain are highly circumscribed. A given occupation is portrayed as a homogeneous group and its work content is objectively defined. As Abbott puts it, public jurisdiction 'assumes exclusive jurisdictions by homogeneous groups. It assumes given tasks without subjective elements' (Abbott 1988: 62).

It is in the legal arena that formal control of work can be conferred. Here, the jurisdictional discourse is even more constrained than in the public domain. All tasks are rigidly defined and boundaries firmly delimited. 'The absolute necessity to abolish all uncertainty leads to a virtually arbitrary definition of the margins of professional jurisdiction' (Abbott 1988: 63). According to Abbott, legal jurisdictions are often uninterpretable in real life situations and this is revealed in the way in which jurisdictional claims are made in the workplace.

According to Abbott, jurisdictional claims in the workplace frequently distort legal boundaries and the public occupational image. Professionals commonly work in complex organisations in which the inter-professional division of labour is frequently replaced by an inter-organisational one. This often leads to a breakdown in inter-professional boundaries, particularly in organisations that are overworked. 'The reality of jurisdictional relations in the workplace is therefore a fuzzy reality indeed' (Abbott 1988: 66). The modern hospital is a case in point.

In early 1993, we were commissioned by South East Thames Regional Health Authority (SETRHA) to undertake a study to investigate the possibilities for expanded nursing role developments in the context of a UK-wide initiative to reduce the hours and improve the working conditions of junior medical staff. At first reading, the research findings appeared to confirm the all-pervasive conservatism amongst doctors and nurses that government ministers have been so keen to emphasise. Nurses, in particular, emerged from the study as resistant to change and in the original study report we considered whether they represented an opposition force with which nurse managers would have to contend in achieving their objectives (Allen *et al.* 1993; Hughes and Allen 1993b). Considered from a sociological perspective, however, these findings may be understood as an interesting window into the processes through which occupations seek to control the parameters of their work and how public and workplace jurisdictional claims intersect. In the following sections we summarise the background to the study, describe some key findings and discuss their sociological significance.

Policy context

Junior Doctors: The New Deal (National Health Service Executive 1991) charged regional health authorities with the task of reducing the excessive hours worked by medical staff. It stipulated that no junior doctor should be working more than 83 hours per week by March 1993 and no more than 72 hours a week by March 1994. Local task forces were established throughout the UK and given the power to recommend the removal of educational approval if standards were not achieved. An increase in the number of career-grade (non-training) posts was called for, along with new ways of organising junior doctors' work, such as the introduction of shift systems. A further suggestion, which is significant for the purposes of this chapter, was the 'sharing' of clinical tasks between nurses and midwives.

The bracketing of nursing role development with junior doctors' hours caused controversy and debate amongst nurses. One US nurse, well known for her writing on the history of the nurse practitioner movement, suggested to us that American nurses would be highly incensed if they were asked to help reduce the hours worked by junior doctors. Indeed, many British nurses protested that they were once again at the 'sharp end' and that doctors were dumping their 'dirty work' on an already overburdened group (Allen and Hughes 1993). Yet, many senior nurse managers, believed that the reduction in junior doctors' hours represented an opportunity for nurses (Directorate of Nursing and Quality SETRHA 1991; Moores 1992; Land *et al.* 1996) and that it was likely to command more resources and managerial support than professionally driven change (Allen and Hughes 1993).

A further catalyst for changes to nursing roles at this time was the publication of *The Scope of Professional Practice* (UKCC 1992). This brought to an end the requirement that nurses, health visitors and midwives needed to gain extended role certificates signed by doctors in order to carry out duties not covered in basic training. In future, responsibility for defining the scope of nursing practice would reside with individual practitioners, providing competency could be demonstrated and role extension did not entail the inappropriate delegation of nursing care to support staff. Supporters of extended nursing roles saw 'the Scope' as a way of freeing nurses from the practice constraints they had faced in the past (e.g. Moores 1992; Ashcroft 1992), whilst others expressed caution and concern that 'traditional nursing values' could be eroded (Hancock 1991; Wright 1995; Clarke 1999). These disagreements are illustrative of much wider tensions within nursing as to the most appropriate route to occupational progression. The delegation of routine medical work to nurses has a long history. As Hughes (1984) has suggested, it is one of the ways in which professions progress. Observing American nursing in the 1950s he concluded that the dropping of low prestige tasks was part of the process by which nursing was becoming a profession.

> As medical technology develops and changes, particular tasks are constantly down-graded; that is, they are delegated by the physician to the nurse. The nurse in turn passes them on to the maid. But occupations and people are being up-graded, within certain limits. The nurse moves up nearer the doctor in techniques and devotes more of her time to the supervision of other workers. The practical nurse is getting more training, and is beginning to insist on the prerogatives which she believes should go with the tasks she performs. New workers come in at the bottom of this hierarchy to take over the tasks abandoned by those occupations which are ascending the mobility ladder. (Hughes 1984: 307–8)

Since this time, however, nurses on both sides of the Atlantic have come to embrace an alternative route to occupational progression reflecting feminist critiques of the professions (see Chapter 1, this volume). Rather than basking in the reflected prestige of medically derived tasks, certain segments of the nursing leadership have been pursuing the claim of autonomous professional status, separate from but equal to medicine. One of the ways in which they have advanced this goal is through the assertion of nursing's unique contribution to the health services division labour which is formulated in terms of a close holistic relationship with patients. Salvage (1988) has coined the phrase 'new nursing' to refer to this alternative professional ideology. As part of this process, tasks which in the past have been downgraded and delegated to support staff – such as physical tending and bedside care – have been reintegrated into the core nursing role. What this reveals, as

Hughes (1984) Jamous and Peloille (1970) and Abbott (1988) have observed, is that the value of an activity is not fixed and may change as a result of other shifts in the system of work. Professionalising processes therefore have to be understood in their historical context. The junior doctors' hours initiative coincided with attempts to restructure nurse education and practice in the UK. The Project 2000 (UKCC 1987) reforms were extensive and have been well-documented in the literature (e.g. Meerabeau 1998). Two issues are crucial for current purposes, however. First, Project 2000 was an explicit professionalising strategy grounded in 'new nursing' ideology. Its aim was to develop a practitioner division of labour based on nurses' 'unique' holistic patient-centred approach to care. As we have seen, under this model of nursing 'basic' tasks such as bathing are given a central place in the qualified nurse's work, and accorded equal importance as supposedly, more scientific or technical tasks handed down to nurses from doctors (Salvage 1992). Second, the proposals entailed a reduction in students' contribution to service provision from 60 to 20 per cent. In the context of rising ministerial concern with healthcare expenditure, the government saw in Project 2000 the possibility for making efficiency savings by modifying the nursing skill mix. In accepting the Project 2000 reforms, the government insisted that the nursing leadership agree to a new support worker – the HCA. This caveat had important implications for the aspirations of the proponents of Project 2000 that all aspects of patient care should be delivered by qualified staff, and soon after its implementation there was evidence of dilution (Ranade 1994: 32). It was against this politically charged backdrop that the study was commissioned.

The study

Nurse managers at SETRHA were broadly supportive of role development. They had already introduced a range of nurse practitioner projects in primary care settings (Directorate of Nursing and Quality, SETRHA 1992) and wished to extend this to the hospital context. The imperative to reduce doctors' hours gave these concerns an added practical impetus. Yet, while the initiative provided a window of opportunity for nurse managers to advance long term objectives, given the debates within the profession as a whole, the reactions of rank-and-file staff were less easy to predict. Against this background, a pilot study was commissioned to explore staff perspectives on expanded nursing roles and their linkage to junior doctors' hours. The research had four major objectives:

(a) to explore the potential for nursing developments in the context of the junior doctors' hours initiative;
(b) to identify how nurses might make a positive contribution to the reduction in junior doctors' hours;
(c) to examine the implications of any changes in the existing division of labour for related occupational groups, that is, auxiliary nurses, HCAs and support workers;
(d) to signpost possible obstacles and barriers to any such initiatives.

Subjects

SETRHA identified eight hospitals within the Region as possible sites for expanded role developments. A questionnaire was prepared to ascertain the views of the occupational groups – junior doctors, nurses, auxiliaries and HCA's[5] – who would be most directly affected. SETRHA established contact with senior nurses at each site to seek their assistance in distributing questionnaires to staff in two wards where expanded developments might shortly be introduced.[6] In the event, five hospitals co-operated in the study. Three hundred and forty-seven questionnaires were distributed and 160 useable completed items were returned, representing a response rate of 46 per cent.

Twelve per cent ($n = 18$) of respondents were auxiliaries or HCAs. Doctors constituted 15 per cent ($n = 23$) of the sample including senior house officers (44 per cent), house officers (17 per cent), registrars (13 per cent), senior registrars (9 per cent), pre-registration house officers (9 per cent) and 'other' (9 per cent). The largest group was qualified nursing staff who comprised 74 per cent ($n = 114$) of the sample. This included C grades (3 per cent), D grades (33 per cent), E grades (37 per cent), F grades (14 per cent), G grades (9 per cent), and 'other' (4 per cent). Eighty-seven per cent of respondents were women and 13 per cent were male. Fifty-one per cent of respondents were aged between 26 and 35 years, 24 per cent between 36 and 50 years, 22 per cent were between 16 and 25 years and only 3 per cent were over 50 years.

The questionnaire

The questionnaire was designed to identify the possibilities and problems of linking expanded nursing role developments to the junior doctors' hours initiative. It covered general attitudes towards expanded roles and junior doctors' hours; the nature of the existing division of labour; utilisation of staff skills and perceived barriers to change. We also included sections aimed at gauging respondents' views on further role developments. We approached this in two ways. One section asked staff to indicate from a list which tasks might be delegated by doctors to nurses and by nurses to support workers. We also attempted to elicit views on six specific expanded role developments (derived from the literature) which were presented in vignette form. As well as requiring conventional forced choice answers, many sections allowed respondents to add more lengthy 'qualitative' comments.

Supplementary data

As a separate background exercise semi-structured telephone interviews were carried out with seven senior nursing officers across the Region, who were asked about the general areas covered in the questionnaire and also provided local contextual information. Several informants suggested useful revisions to the draft questionnaire and assisted in arranging its distribution in their units.

One well-documented methodological difficulty with survey methods is that they inevitably produce a snapshot of complex social phenomena and that they can be notoriously poor predictors of actual behaviour. Moreover, our response rate makes generalisation problematic. Notwithstanding these considerations, however, the nurse managers in the study site regarded the questionnaire as a useful barometer through which to measure the general mood of front-line staff. In this chapter our particular interest is in exploring what these findings reveal about the response of the nursing and medical professions in the study site to a proposal to realign traditional lines of demarcation. In an important sense the responses to our questionnaire represent an opportunity to examine the intersection of the workplace and public jurisdictional claims Abbott (1988) describes. On the one hand, our respondents were grass roots staff familiar with the demands of the work environment and the kinds of informal practices that are frequently necessary to make the system work (see also Chapters 2 and 4, this volume). On the other hand, the questionnaire responses can be regarded as 'public' accounts, oriented as they were to the SETRHA nurse managers and the wider inter-professional political agenda (see also Chapter 3, this volume).

Data analysis

The questionnaire data fell into two categories. Quantitative materials were analysed by computer using the Statistical Package for the Social Sciences (SPSS). Qualitative questionnaire data[7] and telephone interviews were transcribed and categorised on the basis of common themes.

Results

The existing division of labour

A section of the questionnaire was designed to ascertain respondents' opinions of the existing division of labour in their units. Of particular interest were their views of their own role, issues of skill mix and the effects of work pressures on occupational boundaries. Respondents were invited to indicate on a four-point scale their level of agreement with a number of statements.

'I am uncertain as to whether I am allowed to perform certain tasks or not'
These data suggest that the division of labour in the hospitals studied was relatively unambiguous. Fifty-six per cent of respondents maintained that they were rarely uncertain about their roles and responsibilities and 34 per cent said that this was never the case. Analysis of responses revealed no significant differences between occupational groups.

'I perform tasks in my job that I feel unqualified to carry out'
'I perform tasks in my job which are a waste of my time'
Staff claimed that they seldom performed tasks for which they were not qualified: 52 per cent claimed that this was rarely the case and 41 per cent maintained that it was never the case. However, many staff felt that they undertook work that wasted their skills: 5 per cent said they always wasted their skills and 63 per cent claimed that this was often the case. Important differences between the different occupational categories also emerged. About three-quarters of nurses and doctors indicated that their skills were often wasted; yet the picture is reversed for auxiliaries/HCAs, with the same number reporting that their skills were rarely or never wasted.

'I find that doing a job myself is the easiest way of getting things done rather than allocating work according to official job descriptions'
This item was included in the questionnaire because we postulated that the unpredictability of healthcare work would result in a reactive style of work allocation – that is, whoever happens to be faced with a situation deals with it (provided that they have the requisite expertise). The evidence suggests that this frequently applies to doctors: 14 per cent maintained that this was always the case and 60 per cent said it was often the case. Nurses and auxiliaries did not respond conclusively to this item. One possible reason for this is that the work of nurses and ward staff is embedded in the temporal worlds of patients and therefore inherently reactive (see also Chapter 2, this volume). Furthermore, in comparison with doctors their roles are more loosely defined.

The informal division of labour

As we have indicated, observational studies suggest that work pressures and other situational factors may sometimes lead staff to undertake duties which, according to a strict interpretation of the rules, ought to be carried out by another occupational category. Respondents were asked to list those activities (if any) they regularly carried out which transcended their formal work role.

Forty-eight per cent of doctors maintained that they regularly performed activities outside of their role boundaries. The duties referred to were mainly those they believed wasted their time and skills: portering duties, answering telephones, taking results, searching for patients' medical notes and locating and collecting equipment. Some believed that phlebotomy and requesting investigations were also illegitimate functions for medical staff. Somewhat curiously, a few also indicated that prescription of IV fluids was not part of their role. Approximately half the nurse respondents asserted that they performed extra-occupational duties. A large number of nurses complained about administrative duties (filling in forms, answering the telephone, completing investigation request forms, looking for patients' notes and X-rays, and arranging appointments), 'housekeeping' (mopping up spillages, flower arranging, tidying up, re-stocking ward supplies, cleaning) and many also listed domestic duties (filling in patients' menus, distributing meals, making tea and other refreshments).

Some nurses referred to activities others might claim were part of their role, such as washing patients and performing observations of vital signs. Other activities cited lay on the boundary with medicine: for example, giving over-the-counter analgesia before consultation with a doctor, and accepting verbal instructions over the telephone for the administration of medications. A significant number of nurses also listed taking blood, giving intravenous medications and performing cannulation. Most of the extra-occupational tasks nurses claimed that they regularly performed related to the nursing–support worker interface; fewer references were made to tasks at the medical–nursing boundary. Yet, it is only this latter group of activities that nurses believe should be incorporated into the nursing role: respondents suggested that cannulation, venepuncture, filling out request forms, and prescribing certain medications, which are currently performed informally, should come under nurses' formal jurisdiction.

Linking expanded nursing roles and junior doctors' hours

A further section of the questionnaire was designed to ascertain respondents' attitudes to expanded nursing roles, their linkage with the junior doctors' hours initiative and related issues. Respondents were asked to indicate their level of agreement–disagreement with a series of statements based on a five-point scale.

'The need to reduce junior doctors' hours is the concern of doctors and nurses should not be involved in it'
Sixty-four per cent of respondents believed that nurses should make a contribution to the initiative to reduce junior doctors' hours. Seventy-four per cent of doctors and 66 per cent of nurses were in favour of nurses' involvement. There was also a widely held view that nurses would have a tangible impact on the hours worked by doctors. Yet, although 91 per cent of doctors believed that nurses could help to reduce juniors' hours, only 64 per cent of nurses agreed with them.

'The job satisfaction of nurses would be increased by an expansion of nursing duties'
Considered as a group, nurses appeared ambivalent about this issue. Forty-four per cent thought job satisfaction would be improved but 28 per cent did not and 28 per cent adopted a neutral stance.

'By expanding their current duties and responsibilities to include activities traditionally performed by the medical profession nurses would cease to be nurses and become mini-doctors'
The nurses' responses to this item indicated a degree of anxiety about the incorporation of 'medical' tasks into the nursing role. Over half of the nurse respondents pointed to the risk of diluting the nursing role if the traditional scope of practice was expanded, but a further 32 per cent did not consider this to

be a cause for concern. This ambivalence was also evident in the comments made by nurse respondents. Notice how, in the following extract, the respondent contrasts the incorporation of medical work into holistic nursing care (which she favours) with routinised task-allocation.

I would like to carry out expanded roles if it was part of my patient's total nursing care but would not like to be as doctors are at the moment, for example, spending my shift inserting venflons and taking blood.

Doctors, on the other hand, did not share nurses' fears. Sixty-one per cent believed that there was no risk of nurses becoming 'mini-doctors' if they expanded their role. We should note, however, that these findings relate to questions which concerned the *principle* of role expansion and, as we will see in the following sections, compared to nurses, doctors have a rather more circumscribed view of the limits of role expansion. When invited to comment on *specific* expanded role developments (as outlined in vignettes derived from the literature) several medical respondents indicated that they perceived the nursing roles described to be rather too near to the medical end of the healthcare continuum.

'The delegation of medical tasks to nurses will not increase their autonomy and independence in relation to treatment decisions'
More than half of the qualified nurses thought it unlikely that their autonomy would increase as a result of expanded role developments and only 25 per cent believed that it might. Doctors were marginally more optimistic but also ambivalent: 39 per cent thought autonomy would be increased and an equal number maintained that it would not.

'There is no reason why, if nurses get extra training, they cannot make diagnoses and initiate treatments on this basis'
We found only limited support for nurses making diagnostic decisions. Indeed, a great deal of uncertainty surrounds this issue with many respondents taking a neutral/don't know stance. Nurses were actually less enthusiastic than doctors about making diagnoses and initiating treatment: only 33 per cent answered positively to this item and 42 per cent were in disagreement. Forty-four per cent of doctors believed nurses could diagnose and initiate treatment and 39 per cent thought they could not.

'By taking over tasks formerly performed by doctors, nurses will enhance the status of the profession'

Forty-seven per cent of nurses believed that professional status would be enhanced by an expansion of nursing roles, 42 per cent did not and 11 per cent were neutral. Doctors, however, considered the benefits of expanded role developments to the nursing profession to be greater: 70 per cent of doctors claimed that the status of nursing would be enhanced by expanded role developments. These findings indicate interesting differences in the perceived status of work activities between the two occupational groups. The doctors appeared to be operating with a straightforward hierarchy of skills – like the one described by Hughes – with medical tasks at the apex, whereas the nurses were more ambivalent. This is understandable given the debates that were taking place at this time about the appropriate route to occupational progression for nursing.

'Qualified nurses would have too much work to do if they increased their existing activities and responsibilities to include tasks normally performed by doctors'

Although many respondents perceived certain benefits for nurses in expanded role developments, there was also a broadly held view that they would face work-overload if their duties were expanded further: 60 per cent of all respondents maintained that this would be the case, only 19 per cent did not. Unsurprisingly, it was nurses themselves who were most concerned about their onerous workloads: 69 per cent believed expanded nursing roles would create work-overload. Doctors are less convinced: only 36 per cent of doctors believed nurses would have too much to do and 45 per cent maintained that they would not.

'If qualified nurses expand their current activities health care assistants will need to take over some of the tasks normally performed by qualified staff'

Although the different occupational groups disagreed about the implications of expanded roles for nurses' workload, there was a broad consensus that it would necessitate the devolution of certain 'nursing' tasks to auxiliaries/HCAs. Seventy-seven per cent of respondents believed that this would be the case; little variation was found between the different occupational groups.

Yet, there was also a widely held view (66 per cent) that HCAs lack the theoretical knowledge to extend their activities beyond their current duties. Nurses expressed most reservations about the ability of HCAs to expand their scope of practice: 73 per cent did not consider that HCAs/auxiliaries possessed a knowledge-base that would allow them to do this. HCAs/auxiliaries were rather more confident about their ability to expand their remit but this was by no means unanimous: 47 per cent believed they had sufficient knowledge and 29 per cent did not. Considerable uncertainty existed on this issue amongst medical staff: 35 per cent thought their knowledge to be sufficient, 44 per cent believed it was not and 22 per cent were uncertain.

Options for the future division of labour

In one section of the questionnaire we asked respondents to study a list of tasks and to indicate which of these could be delegated from doctors to nurses and which from nurses to HCAs.

The medical–nursing interface

Doctors and nurses agree on certain activities that could be performed by nurses (Table 5.1) and those which could not (Table 5.2).

However, our survey revealed an area of middle ground where a tension existed between the duties doctors *wanted* to delegate and those nurses were *prepared* to take on and those duties nurses *wanted* to take on and those doctors were *prepared* to devolve (Table 5.3).

One underlying trend in the responses to this section of the questionnaire is that, on the whole, nurses were rather more cautious about assuming 'medical' tasks than doctors were about delegating them. Even where both groups agreed that a task could and should be delegated, support tended to be more muted from nurses. Nurses, however, were rather more enthusiastic about increasing their involvement in the social dimensions of patient care – through, history taking, for example – but doctors were less than happy to delegate these activities. There were also indications of resistance from within

Table 5.1 Agreement on activities that can be performed by nurses.

Task	Percentage of respondents who agree task *can* be delegated to nurses
Obtaining venous blood	89
Inserting intravenous cannulae	86
Performing electrocardiographs	96
Prescription of anti-emetics	76
Prescription of laxatives	92
Prescription of evacuant enemata	89
Prescription of night sedation	76
Prescription of 'over-the-counter' analgesia	89
Removal of a chest drain	74
Percussion of the urinary bladder for distension	89
Performing defibrillation	75
Administration of intravenous analgesia	91
Administration of intravenous antibiotics	98
Administration of intravenous chemotherapy	81
Initiation and performance of urinary catheterisation of male patients	71
Urinary catheterisation of male patients	75
Independently ordering laboratory investigations	73

Table 5.2 Agreement on activities that cannot be performed by nurses.

Task	Percentage of respondents who agree task *cannot* be delegated to nurses
Prescriptions of medications for chronic illness	59
Initiation and performance of a pleural tap	90
Performance of a pleural tap	90
Initiation and removal of a chest drain	60
Initiation and performance of a bone-marrow biopsy	97
Performance of a bone-marrow biopsy	95
Initiation and performance of a lumbar puncture	97
Performance of a lumbar puncture	95
Examination of the eyes with an opthalmascope	61
Initiation and performance of intubation	64
Obtaining arterial blood	65
Conducting a review of body systems	66

Table 5.3 Trend in response to a questionnaire on the kinds of 'medical' tasks that nurses can undertake.

Task	Percentage of nurses who think nurses can undertake the activity	Percentage of doctors who think nurses can undertake the activity
Obtain a patient's consent to surgical procedures	36	52
Confirm the death of a patient	59	86
Making discharge decision	42	17
Summarise a patient's past medical history	72	57
Obtain a history of the patient's current illness	70	48

both occupational groups to nurses taking independent action on the basis of a diagnosis. For example, although 96 per cent of respondents thought nurses should perform ECGs, only 24 per cent believed they should be able to initiate an ECG, interpret the results and start treatment. There were similar findings with respect to defibrillation.

The nursing–HCA interface

Nurses and auxiliaries were asked to indicate from a list of tasks those they believed could be performed by an auxiliary (if appropriate training were given). As with the nurses and doctors, there were certain activities that both groups agreed could be devolved to auxiliaries or HCAs (Table 5.4) and others that they agreed could not (Table 5.5).

There were a number of activities which auxiliaries/HCAs believed they could undertake but nurses felt cautious about delegating (Table 5.6).

Similar tensions existed in relation to the delegation of suture removal, clip removal, drain removal and the re-stocking of emergency equipment. There was not one area that nurses wished to delegate which auxiliaries were unhappy to

Table 5.4 Activities that can be devolved to auxiliaries or HCAs.

Task	Percentage of respondents who believe the task can be delegated to auxiliaries/HCAs
Catheter care	93
Measuring and recording blood pressure	86
Measuring and recording blood sugar	80
Measuring peak flow	87
Accompanying patients with intravenous infusions to other hospital departments	75
Administration of evacuant enema	68
Removal of intravenous cannulae	68
Administration of evacuant suppositories	89
Removal of a nasogastric tube	70
Pre-operative shaves	97
Taking a swab	74
Collection of blood from blood bank	95
Collection of controlled drugs from pharmacy	74
Preparation of a trolley and equipment for sterile procedures	73
Obtaining catheter specimen of urine	94

Table 5.5 Activities that cannot be devolved to auxiliaries or HCAs.

Task	Percentage of respondents who think the task cannot be delegated to auxiliaries/HCAs
Administration of intravenous medications	93
Administration of intramuscular medications	89
Passing a nasogastric tube	72
Removal of sutures	67
Removal of clips	68
Removal of wound drains	76

undertake. Qualitative data derived from the comments section of the questionnaire suggested that nurses believed that rather than delegating work to auxiliaries/HCAs extra qualified staff would be needed if nurses were to extend their role.

If nurses are going to expand their duties, then there must be more qualified nurses, rather than increasing HCAs' responsibilities. Also the grading of staff should reflect their duties.

If nurses take on these extra responsibilities it is essential that they receive adequate appropriate training. Also they will need to relinquish some of their other roles to unqualified staff, which is not satisfactory. It would be more appropriate to increase the number of nursing qualified staff to enable them to provide *total* patient care for a *smaller* group of patients. Increasing the number of HCAs would only be a cheap way out. The ultimate responsibility for care that patients' receive lies with the qualified nurse and it is therefore she who would feel pressurised.

Table 5.6   Disagreement on the activities that can be delegated.

Task	Percentage of auxiliaries/HCAs who think the task can be delegated	Percentage of nurses who think the task can be delegated
Redress wound	60	37
Administer oral medications	69	30
Measure and record neurological observations	69	37

Specific expanded role developments: the vignettes

In addition to the task lists, we also sought respondents' views on six specific expanded role developments described in the literature and which were summarised in the questionnaire in the form of short vignettes. These comprised:

- *Admissions Nurse Practitioner*   Nurses perform all the preliminary stages of the patient's admission to hospital – they obtain a history of the current illness and relevant social and past medical history, initiate laboratory tests and order X-rays according to protocols. When the doctor first encounters the patient many of the details and information necessary to make a provisional diagnosis and commence treatment will be available.
- *Accident and Emergency Nurse Practitioner*   In accident and emergency departments selected nurse practitioners

function in an independent capacity, attending to minor cases – for example, suturing minor lacerations, removing foreign bodies, prescribing medications (according to protocols) – the patient never having to see the physician unless referral is necessary.

● *Surgeon's Assistant* Nurse practitioners work as surgeon's assistants in operating theatres. Nurses functioning in this capacity teach and prepare patients pre-operatively, obtain their consent, assist the surgeon with the operation, closing wounds and performing minor surgical procedures.

● *Accident and Emergency Trauma Specialist Nurse* Trauma specialist nurses in accident and emergency departments function in an expanded role in the care of seriously ill patients. Nurses evaluate a patient's injury, make a diagnosis and act on this basis. Nurses' domain of clinical practice includes: insertion of intravenous and central venous pressure catheters, intubation, drawing arterial blood gases, auscultation for breath and bowel sounds, interpretation of X-rays and laboratory results. In the absence of the presence of the physician the trauma nurse relies on her knowledge of physiology and trauma in exercising judgement in managing the patient.

● *Outpatient Nurse Practitioner* Nurse practitioners in out-patient departments have responsibility for the maintenance and management of patients with chronic disorders. Nurse practitioners carry their own caseload, advise on aspects of living with a chronic disorder, modify and prescribe medication regimens, make referrals to other agencies and function in a supportive capacity. Patients are referred to the physician as necessary.

● *Paediatric Nurse Practitioner* The paediatric nurse practitioner diagnoses and manages certain commonly encountered conditions according to protocols. The nurse obtains the medical and social history and performs an initial physical examination. The nurse may intervene directly with the critically ill newborn. In the event of an emergency condition the practitioner resuscitates and treats the infant with such procedures as endotracheal intubation, vessel catheterisation, thoracentesis and the use of certain medications. The nurse can also insert umbilical catheters, draw venous and arterial blood samples, and perform bladder aspiration. The nurse has additional skills in the domain of ordering and interpreting laboratory tests and certain emergency X-rays, and in the counselling of parents. Nurses care for critically ill neonates during transport to hospital.

On the whole, nurses tended to be more enthusiastic about these holistic role developments than they were about discrete task delegation, whereas doctors' enthusiasm for the expanded roles described in this section was muted. Doctors perceived the main beneficiaries of holistic role developments to be nurses rather than doctors or patients. Nurses, by contrast, stressed the benefits for patient care. Although both doctors and nurses greet different roles with varying degrees of enthusiasm, there was a widespread belief that implementation of all these innovations would be hampered by lack of nursing time, the need for additional staff and insufficient resources for additional training.

There was most support for expanded role developments in ambulatory settings: that is, the outpatient nurse practitioner and the accident and emergency nurse practitioner.

Respondents believed that these roles would reduce junior doctors' hours and would increase nurses' job satisfaction and would have no deleterious effect on standards of patient care. In fact, a substantial majority (64 per cent) claimed that nurse practitioners in outpatient departments would actually lead to improvements in patient care.

There was rather less support for those expanded role developments which entailed nurses undertaking complex 'technical' tasks: that is, the paediatric nurse practitioner, trauma accident and emergency nurse practitioner and the surgeon's assistant roles. Although respondents felt that they would decrease junior doctors' hours and augment nurses' job satisfaction, there was widespread concern about the likely effects on standards of patient care. A majority indicated that there were significant barriers to the implementation of these roles. Doctors were particularly sceptical.

If nurses want to play at doctor then they should go to medical school. (Doctor commenting on the Accident and Emergency Trauma Specialist Vignette)

Why not become a surgeon? That's the job. (Doctor commenting on the Surgeon's Assistant Vignette)

We found moderate support for the admissions nurse practitioner role, although doctors were less enthusiastic than nursing staff. One objection raised is that in taking a history doctors employ highly individualised methodologies, and that many doctors would insist on repeating this process with their patients in order to reach a diagnosis, thereby creating repetition.

Barriers to change

One section of our questionnaire was designed to ascertain perceived barriers to change. Respondents were asked to indicate from a list the four most important barriers to change in rank order. Unfortunately, a significant proportion of respondents failed to complete this section correctly by ranking barriers in order of importance: instead they simply indicated four (unranked) barriers to change. We have therefore been forced to opt for a more basic mode of analysis than planned: responses were accumulated and the four most often cited barriers were identified. The most important barriers to change as perceived by the sample population as a whole are listed in Table 5.7

There were some interesting differences in the barriers perceived by the various occupational groups. An important barrier for qualified nursing staff was that of 'too few nurses to function in an expanded role': this was identified by 79.0 per cent of qualified nurses and supported by many of the comments made by respondents.

Table 5.7 Perceived barriers to change.

Barrier to change	Percentage of respondents selecting this item
Unclear lines of accountability	79
Too few nurses to function satisfactorily in an expanded role	69
Legal restrictions	61
The need to undertake further training	51

It's all very well reducing doctors' hours (and I am in agreement with it). However, would nursing manpower (sic) increase?

Whilst doctors conceded that the lack of nursing staff was an obstacle to change they did not perceive this problem as keenly as nursing staff: 42 per cent of doctors selected this item. Doctors (60 per cent) indicated that the 'unwillingness of nurses to take on the responsibilities of a new role was an important obstacle to such developments. But nurses did not share this view: only 25 per cent believed that this constituted a barrier to change. The most frequently cited barrier to change given by auxiliaries/HCAs (72 per cent) was 'legal restrictions'. Fifty-four per cent of qualified nurses agreed but doctors did not. Yet, as we have seen, the latter had a more circumscribed conception of the principle of expanded role developments – for them, delegation meant the passing down of tasks but not the associated decision-making. Moreover, we suggest that legal restrictions will seem a more formidable barrier to change for those lower down the occupational hierarchy where the limitations of one's role are reinforced on a daily basis by reference to legal jurisdictional monopolies. Our respondents also indicated concern about organisational accountability. This was seen as the most significant barrier to change by both nurses and doctors and ranked second with HCAs/auxiliaries. Many respondents added comments stressing the need for clear guidelines for practice and the development of clinical protocols to safeguard staff.

Discussion: barriers to change or jurisdictional claims making

Our findings indicate that all three occupational groups shared the view that nurses should be involved in developments to reduce the hours worked by junior doctors. Doctors and nurses, and nurses and auxiliaries also agreed on a range of tasks that could be delegated, and considerable support was found for specific expanded role developments such as outpatient nurse practitioners and accident and emergency nurse practitioners. Yet, despite this wide measure of consensus regarding the positive potential of expanded roles, there were also clear areas of tension and disagreement between the various stake-holders. Doctors were willing to delegate many of their traditional tasks to nurses, but nurses were less enthusiastic about accepting certain of them. Auxiliaries/HCAs were eager to expand their existing work domain, but nurses were reluctant to delegate certain aspects of their work. Nurses were also particularly cautious about role change. A large number indicated that they thought the distinctive nursing role would be endangered if traditional medical tasks were incorporated into it.

I feel many selected and specially trained nurses could do a lot of doctors' work and probably in a kinder way – however – I feel that ability is not what we should be talking about and is quite different to eroding the profession of nursing, and having time to perform the *nursing* role really well i.e. listening to the patient, using counselling skills, educating, discharge planning, nursing procedures, observations, some 'hands-on' specialist care etc.

I believe that patients have a right to the best possible nursing care from a *trained named* nurse. [...] and similarly the right to a doctor to assess, prescribe and give medical care. Some overlap – yes – but take care. Highly specialised nurses trained in some of the areas suggested really wouldn't be nurses any more. When non-nurses give care that really should be given by trained nurses – it could mean the end of the nursing profession. I agree with change and growth of the profession – but I don't think being mini-doctors is an enhancement of our profession necessarily.

There was also a widely held view that expanded role developments would not enhance nurses' autonomy and independence in relation to treatment decisions, and considerable uncertainty was expressed as to whether there were any benefits to be gained for nurses either in terms of their job satisfaction or their professional status. There was also a widespread belief that an expansion of the nursing role would result in work overload.

Nurses often or all too frequently take on other people's jobs, e.g. portering, catering, medical tasks, which HCAs ought to be able to do but can't and domestic work. We are not paid extra for doing this but we do it because if we didn't who would? At the end of the day it is the patient who suffers...nurses are, and always have been willing to improve their skills but we are not here to relieve doctors' workloads when we have already got so much to do.

You can't make the assumption that because nurses are the largest group of staff that they are the sponge for every additional duty.

Moreover, while autonomy figured prominently in the public jurisdictional claims of the nursing leadership, our findings also indicate that amongst grass-roots staff there is concern about the legal implications of expanded roles and organisational accountability. Although the new UKCC guidelines have been heralded by many as recognition of the professionalism of nurses, they leave many nurses feeling vulnerable (also see, Dowling 1997). The onus of expanded practice remains with the individual nurse (acting in accord with the UKCC Code of Professional Conduct, and an implicit model of professional autonomy). Yet, in reality, the limits of autonomy in a managed service are all too apparent (also see, Salvage 1992; Dowling *et al.* 1996).

Nurses' responses also indicated a strong belief in the need for additional qualified staff rather than more support workers. Many expressed the view that support staff did not have adequate knowledge to extend their existing roles and responsibilities.

I believe that any responsible, intelligent individual could be *trained* to do *all* of the listed activities. However I *do not believe* that 'training' necessarily implies education about and/or comprehension of the many complexities implied in either the actual decision to perform a given task or the interpretation of outcomes, good or bad. [...] Training to perform these activities is easy to provide. However I was *educated* as a nurse not just to carry out such tasks but also to understand the significance of a multiplicity of nursing observations which I now make whilst carrying out the tasks.

But while our respondents appeared to have genuine concerns about the effects of 'dilution' on standards of patient care there were other contrary trends in their responses. For example, despite a reluctance to delegate many tasks to auxiliaries/HCAs, a significant number of nurses do support the delegation of 'basic nursing care' activities (see also Clarke 1999). One possible explanation for these apparently contradictory findings is that they reflect wider tensions within nursing between 'new nursing' ideologies in which basic care is highly valued, and traditional skill hierarchies in which it is devalued and delegated in the search of efficiency. It may also reflect underlying strains between the professional ideals of nursing staff and their public jurisdictional claims and the reality of service demands. Study after study has shown that despite the professional rhetoric, qualified nurses rarely perform bedside care in practice because of the demands of the work setting (Buckenham and McGrath 1983; Melia 1987; Allen 2001a). Although nurses tended to be more conservative than doctors in respect of the delegation of tasks, doctors were more cautious than nurses were when specific *roles* were considered. It was nurses who tended to favour specific holistic role developments. We suggest that these divergent views reflect the respective professional interests of the two occupational groups. The medical profession has always jealousy protected its power and prestige, and arguably this is threatened less by the devolution of discrete tasks to nurses than it is by holistic expanded role developments which may entail the delegation of decision-making to nurses. Similarly, the professional agenda of nursing which aims to establish a domain of practice based on a claim to a unique holistic approach to care is more congruent with holistic role developments. First, in their public jurisdictional claims nurses have tended to emphasise their contribution to healthcare that distinguishes nursing from medicine, rather than emphasising areas of overlap. Second, our findings indicate that many nurses feared that embracing discrete medical tasks in the absence of additional nursing staff would create a strain towards task allocation and result in the need to delegate 'nursing' activities to support staff.

It would seem that cost-containment concerns within the NHS have generated significant scepticism amongst staff as to the availability of resources for new initiatives. If we consider this alongside nursing's professionalising aims and its occupational history then it should come as no surprise that the nursing response to a management-led initiative should be cautious. So, while it is true that nurses were most wary about changes to the status quo, this should not be overstated. Arguably this hesitancy had good foundation. The structure of interest is such that nurses perceived many of the developments we explored to be of little immediate benefit to them. The advantages to doctors, in terms of reduced hours, and to auxiliaries, in terms of job satisfaction, were altogether more apparent.

Given these findings it would be all too easy to conclude that it is nurses who are the conservative force in the change process. Yet, this view is simply not borne out by the empirical evidence. Since the last century the content of nursing work has been in a permanent state of flux, fashioned and refashioned by competing pressures such as the labour requirements of the healthcare institutions, the demands of doctors for skilled assistance, and the desire of nurses to increase the autonomy, satisfaction and status of their work. Profoundly affected by gender ideologies that devalue care, service needs have tended to be the most decisive factors when nursing policy is made (Beardshaw and Robinson 1990). In actuality there have been widespread nursing role developments since *The New Deal* was first introduced and the furore, which characterised the professional debates at the time of our study have subsided. There now appears to be a degree of resignation that the medical–nursing boundary has shifted – in some areas permanently (UKCC 1999a) – and attention has now refocused on the issue of how the plethora of posts and titles which have evolved in the wake of the junior doctors' hours initiative and the *Scope of Professional Practice* (UKCC 1992) should be regulated and standards safeguarded (UKCC 1999a,b).

At the time of writing role change is once again on the agenda. Junior doctors' hours are being revisited in order to bring them in line with the European working time directive (Department of Trade & Industry 1999)[8] and recent policy trends signal a strong move towards the breakdown of traditional lines of demarcation (Department of Health 2000a). These developments are bound to stir more public and professional debate and expressions of resistance from the professions concerned. Far from seeing this as representing some kind of built-in conservatism amongst the health occupations, however, we should understand this as an expression of the micro-political processes through which occupations evolve and develop. In other words, resistance to change is a *normal* part of jurisdictional claims-making.

6 Continuing professional education and the everyday realities of practice

Sue Jordan and David Hughes

Introduction

This chapter is concerned with the relationship between continuing professional education (CPE) and organisational change. It utilises data from two studies of nurses returning to practice after completing advanced bioscience courses to examine some of the barriers to change that they encountered, and their perceptions of how their enhanced skills might affect their roles. In line with the wider aims of this book, the chapter reinforces the argument that roles and role change need to be understood within the context of the wider ecology of the organisation, including the existing division of labour, work cultures and patterns of authority relations.

There is a tendency to see CPE as a self-contained, monoprofessional exercise which can change practice by improving the individual competencies of practitioners. Usually, CPE is not co-ordinated with any wider set of initiatives aimed at changing the work settings from which students are drawn, and – in most cases – there is no equivalent preparation for co-workers from other disciplines, or necessarily even the same discipline. Recent years have seen a rapid expansion of CPE provision, particularly in nursing. However, although CPE is a burgeoning industry, its impact remains unclear. While there is an abundant and proliferating literature describing course developments, empirical data on practice changes and clinical outcomes are thin on the ground. For example, in a systematic review of 102 trials of interventions designed to enhance the performance of healthcare professionals, Oxman (1994) was able to identify only 12 studies evaluating the impact of educational initiatives on professional performance. The individualised focus of CPE tends to carry across into the few studies that have sought to chart its impact. By focusing on the application of knowledge to the minutiae of daily care, some authors have linked classroom input to practice outcomes (Cox and Baker 1981; Foglesong *et al.* 1987; Meservy and Monson 1987; Alexander 1990; Brooker *et al.* 1994). However, most of these studies are based either on single outcome measures (Davis *et al.* 1992, 1995) or 'chart audit' (Cox and Baker 1981; Meservy and Monson 1987; Waddell 1991). 'Proxy' measures of effectiveness, such as prescribing patterns or laboratory test uptakes, are only relevant to certain aspects of care, and are dependent on the accuracy and accessibility of medical records or databases (Kanouse and Jacoby 1988). The difficulty with the 'chart audit' approach is that improvements in patients' records may not necessarily translate into improved care delivery. It is also the case that many studies of this genre have failed to identify any improvements in care attributable to CPE (McClosky 1981; Hutton 1987; Dunn *et al.* 1988; Lima-Bastow 1995; de Burgh *et al.* 1995; Bradley *et al.* 1997).

It could be argued that the individualised focus of CPE initiatives, as well as the associated evaluations, results in the neglect of a whole range of contextual factors that affect practice change. For example, we know from the extensive literature on the 'theory/practice gap' that academic nursing has faced recurrent problems in gaining acceptance for its ideas and prescriptions for change in real practice settings. While the gap has often been attributed to the limited applicability of academic knowledge to the practice situation, many writers also point to attitudinal factors and the organisational contexts of clinical settings. Thus, there has been much discussion of the role of work hierarchies and traditional attitudes (Bircumshaw 1989; Carlisle 1991; Kelly 1996), the persistence of routine and ritual (Craddock 1993), workload pressures (Ogier 1989), the complexities of implementing the new forms of nurse education (Rafferty *et al.* 1996), and the significance of bureaucratic structures (Hewison and Wildman 1996; Heslop *et al.* 2001).

Resources and funding arrangements, the lead set by management and the stance of co-workers seem particularly important factors affecting practice changes. Audit suggests that changes in patient care are more likely to be attributable to financial incentives than education programmes (Kristiansen and Holtedahl 1993; Robinson 1994; Rittenhouse 1994; Howie *et al.* 1994; Stelfox 1998). Organisational constraints, such as time, staff shortages and turnover, workload, and emergency situations also impede the transfer of knowledge to practice (Francke *et al.* 1995; Meservy and Monson 1987). Where staff morale is low, resistance to graduates' initiatives to change outdated practice may be pronounced and even threatening (Ewens *et al.* 2001). The issue of managerial and collegial support has figured centrally in a number of studies (Foglesong *et al.* 1987; Brooker and Butterworth 1991; Scheller 1993; Nolan *et al.* 1995). Managers may find supporting graduates in clinical innovations difficult within their limited resources, and without policy directives or guidance (Brooker *et al.* 1994). However, where older studies report negative attitudes in the workplace towards graduates of both pre- and post-registration programmes (e.g. Bircumshaw 1989; Carlisle 1991; Kelly 1996), more recent work in settings where graduate nurses were more numerous found more ambivalent attitudes (Dowswell *et al.* 1998; Jordan and Hughes 1998).

This paper presents data from two linked research projects that were consciously designed to have a wider focus, including both the clinical outcomes of CPE and the influence of the wider organisational environment. However, both were exploratory studies, the first with a wider focus and the second a smaller scale project, and were intended to pave the way for a larger study. Consequently, the findings should be regarded as hypotheses to be tested via further research rather than as the last word on these issues. The findings relating to clinical outcomes have been published elsewhere (Jordan and Reid 1997; Jordan 1998; Jordan and Hughes 1998; Jordan *et al.* 1999; Jordan and Hughes 2000), and this chapter is concerned mainly with the organisational dimension.

The research

The two studies considered here investigated the impact of post-registration nursing courses, and were both undertaken by teams led by Jordan. The first study examined a part-time applied physiology course, leading to a Diploma in Nursing qualification, where students came from all branches of the health service. It centred on a single cohort of nurses ($n = 42$) who came from diverse practice areas including medical, surgical, elderly care, mental health and community nursing. This course was designed to apply the foundations of physiology to the delivery of patient care, and to equip students with advanced bioscience knowledge with potential applicability to areas of practice such as: standardising BP readings, assessing dehydration, monitoring pain and its cardiovascular consequences, and introducing temperature monitoring. The study aimed to assess the success of the course in achieving its objective of transmitting practice-relevant knowledge to students. Nurses' views of the course and its impact on practice were explored using three methods. Students were required to keep academic diaries over a six-month period and record examples where the course had affected their work practices (which continued alongside their academic studies). A questionnaire was completed before and after the course. Finally, after course completion, in-depth qualitative interviews were carried out with 25 per cent of the cohort.

The second study focused on a specialist pharmacology module for community mental health nurses (CMHNs). It examined the impact on the clinical practice of CMHNs who completed the course, in relation to a comparator group (Jordan *et al.* 1999). The course aimed to equip CMHNs to monitor patients for the side effects of prescribed medication, and the research was designed to investigate how far this took place. Students were seconded from their employment to study full-time for one year, and then returned to their former practice areas. Again, a mixed method approach was used, this time combining interviews and questionnaires with non-participant observation of clinical practice. Data were collected on the experiences of a single cohort of students ($n = 7$) and an equal number of matched comparators before the course, after the course and six months later. The comparators had not undertaken post-registration education in pharmacology and were matched in terms of work experience and location.

This later study aimed to address certain questions that had not been resolved by the initial investigation. The first study had shown that most students valued the new knowledge that the course had imparted and that most claimed to apply this in their practice. However, it gave little indication of the extent to which the new knowledge was utilised by all nurses, and provided no independent verification of the accuracy of the students' self-reports of their behaviours. The second study was constructed to rectify these shortcomings by including direct observation of nurses at work and narrowing the focus to a single practice area where the impact of CPE could be more precisely monitored.

As indicated above, the present chapter is concerned with the subset of findings about CPE and the implementation of change in the face of organisational constraints. It relies mainly on data from qualitative interviews, supported by background observations of nurses at work. In the sections that follow we first consider respondents' accounts of three factors that placed major constraints on change: lack of time and resources, opposition from nursing colleagues and opposition from doctors. We then discuss nurses' perceptions of the purpose and benefits of CPE, highlighting the limited nature of their aspirations and their reluctance to challenge the existing order. Here, we look at nurses' reluctance to 'police' the doctors, their lack of enthusiasm for nurse prescribing, and their tendency to equate CPE with occupational survival rather than career advancement.

Time and resources

Although there was some evidence that clinical practice had changed to accommodate course objectives, the barriers to change were sometimes overwhelming. The most frequently cited barrier to change was resource constraints. The incorporation of the knowledge gained in CPE into practice may be proportional to the staff/patient ratio (Foglesong *et al.* 1987). For example, in the second study, we found that the CMHNs with the highest caseloads reported greater difficulties in changing practice. Some students felt that they were unable to apply the knowledge gained from the course due to lack of time, and the demands made on the service. This meant that nursing pharmacology was accorded a low priority. More than one respondent described a service in crisis:

> It's because I've got so much of everything to do [...] The girls in our office are very stressed because of the actual numbers of patients. One of my colleagues feels that she isn't working effectively because of the numbers she has got [on her caseload] – 70 or 80 something. [...] The ambulances can't take on referrals to transport people to day care at the moment. They are at saturation. Home Care can't take referrals because they are full, so people can't have basic services. People who can't afford to pay for a private agency are having major problems, so we make inappropriate and too many referrals to our own team, who in turn are overworked and over-stretched. [...] We just keep thinking that perhaps things will be better in April, because Home Care will take referrals again then and social services will take on referrals, but they just stop in October and nobody gets Home Care. [...] Everything is beyond our control, that's the difficult thing, when you are the main person going into somebody's home and you recognise somebody desperately needs help and you can't give it and yet they are looking to you to sort something, it's hard and worrying. (CMHN, working with older people, 6 months post-course)

This suggests that the educational effectiveness of the courses was limited by resource constraints and service funding. Some respondents felt that the need for practice change was dwarfed by overwhelming problems of staffing and other resources. Changes in service provision, even at the level of specialty policies, often require a redistribution of resources over which CPE has no influence. Only where the course objectives were congruent with the priorities of senior doctors or managers, did practice change.

Senior nurses as a barrier to change

The stance of organisational superiors can be a critical factor in promoting or impeding role changes affecting rank-and-file staff. Respondents in both studies reported that it was senior nurses, not doctors, who were the most significant barrier to changes in clinical practice. Indeed, this accords with the findings of several previous investigations (Jacono and Jacono 1994; Nolan *et al.* 1995; Miller 1995; Lemp 1995). Respondents had strong views about the attitude taken by senior nursing colleagues when they returned from their training:

> I gained. The ward didn't. They wouldn't use my knowledge to full advantage. They could have got more value from the course [...] Frustration is an understatement. It's some nurses. The doctor is approachable. Long stay patients and long stay staff – they feel threatened. It's the: 'There's no point' attitude. (Senior staff nurse, hospital for mentally ill older people)

Many respondents believed that senior nurses, who did not themselves possess qualifications in bioscience, saw the diploma nurses as a threat to their own authority and expertise. Individual nurses reported a sense of isolation and lack of support from senior colleagues.

> The nursing hierarchy are the worst. There's rocking the boat with excessive knowledge. A lot of nurses give up because of this [...] Frustration increases when you can't change things. You can only bang your head for so long. Nurses themselves are stopping things, especially areas like wound care. (Specialist nurse, ulcer clinic)

> The hierarchy are threatened – it's: 'Who does she think she is?' They're not interested in change. Attitudes are the biggest problem [...] The old school nurses are the worst. The others want to learn. (Sister, coronary care)

This lack of support from senior colleagues meant that the extent of role change was limited. Individual nurses could improve their own practice in areas such as standardised blood pressure monitoring, for example, by using a defined diastolic end point and incorporating orthostatic assessment. However, only the most senior nurses were able to update policies on BP monitoring in their clinical areas. Systematic changes in practice required managerial support, which was not always forthcoming. A majority of CMHNs completing the bioscience course agreed that managers and senior colleagues constituted a barrier to change. Four out of seven students said they found them unsupportive. Some CMHNs reported similar entrenched attitudes from senior colleagues. But in the second study we found considerable variation amongst respondents. Four students had found managers and colleagues unsupportive, but two respondents (one student, one comparator) said there was no opposition from other nurses. One of the main complaints was that, while superiors paid lip service to the value of continuing professional education, they were all too ready to dismiss the knowledge gained as 'academic' and inapplicable to real practice.

> I have increased awareness about certain aspects of my work, which are important, and I don't have the time to implement or develop. I feel that I am not doing my clients justice, or myself maybe. It's frustration more than anything. You gain new knowledge, and you can't really do anything with it, and other people are not really interested or they take the **** out of you because you have 'gone all academic'. It's *my* job, I'm trying to do my job better than I did before so that's hard. [...] They're not interested at all. [...] The managers in theory go for it, but with regard to practical support, as in time or space, not really. And I think other colleagues aren't particularly interested because they are all in the same boat, everyone feels overworked and undervalued and people don't want to take on any more, or they can't. (CMHN, 6 months post-course)

The perception that managers will not let nurses use their new knowledge is also evident in the following quotation from a comparator mental health nurse, who links this to more general doubts about whether the acquisition of such knowledge is worthwhile.

> Knowledge is all very well, but it's more trouble than the worth of it. The wards take no notice. Managers and charge nurses won't discuss things. They are more likely to do something if you say it's for your project, rather than just for 'the good of the patient'. [...] They're still bandaging [lower leg ulcers] from the top down. They aren't even certain whether the ulcer is venous or arterial. [...] We are not getting knowledge for our patients' benefit, but for our own promotion. (Comparator student)

Two CMHNs gave more ambiguous responses, suggesting only that lack of support from colleagues might be a problem, in one case indirectly because of workload pressures.

> Perhaps I should hedge my bets and say it should be a team initiative. Perhaps it shouldn't come from any one specific group because you are looking at team interventions. [...] If nothing is going to change it's a pointless exercise I suppose. It's probably not going to happen unless I am pushed a bit. (CMHN, 6 months post-course)

> I wouldn't say there would be a problem here because the consultant and manager feel very committed to the seriously mentally ill, but I guess there could be a problem in time if you have a heavy workload. (CMHN, immediately post-course)

The remaining respondent completing the course stated that she anticipated no opposition from superiors in her clinical area.

Higher education may render nurses less amenable to control by their seniors (Castledine 1992; Perry 1995), making nursing management feel threatened. Sometimes the nurse managers' opposition to new patterns of working is accentuated by a lack of resources for what they see as basic nursing work (for comparison, see Brooker *et al.* 1994). In response, they cause frustration by thwarting change (Nolan *et al.* 1995; Francke *et al.* 1995). It might be supposed that the scope for open opposition to nurses' possession of biomedical knowledge has been undermined by the *de facto* introduction of nurse prescribing, and the proposals contained in the second *Crown Report* (Department of Health 1999). However, it seems that some senior nurses continue to engage in more covert forms of resistance, which can damage the morale of those completing advanced courses.

Medical opposition

Both studies found that doctors had mixed reactions to the nurses' increased knowledge. Generally, the picture emerging from the data is consistent with previous research which suggests that younger doctors are more receptive to nurses' suggestions, but, with time and growing experience, become more socially distant so that nurses have to be more circumspect and deferential in their attempts to exert influence (Burling *et al.* 1956; Mauksch 1996; Light 1975; Devine 1978; Hughes 1988). Several nurses reported instances when doctors were supportive when they used their expanded bioscience knowledge.

> To have physiological knowledge is so important – a gentleman with Parkinson's and bilateral fractures developed contractures. I applied my physiology. The L-dopa was wasted at lunch and teatime. I spoke to the doctor to re-time the medications. She told me to check with pharmacy first. After two days the 'Physio' noticed the improvement. The staff felt positive. The team shared the knowledge. Another nurse will think of this. It teaches us to act as patients' advocates, to ask for medication review. (Staff nurse, trauma unit)

However, there were also many examples of tension and conflict.

> They don't always know best. Two weeks ago I asked for an admission for assessment. They refused. That meant that treatment for a strangulated hernia was delayed. (CMHN)
>
> They'll do their own thing anyway: 'You're just a nurse. I'm the doctor.' That's it at the end of the day. (Junior staff nurse, dermatology ward)
>
> The doctors are a barrier, now I'm better informed. Inappropriate ADH [anti-diuretic hormone] secretion post-op now. This wasn't as isolated as I'd thought. It's a common mistake [...] I challenged the doctor. His response was: 'You're going to become a doctor'. (Sister, surgical unit)

Such accounts echo Fairman's (1992) description of nurses being accused of 'playing doctor' (see also Chapter 5, this volume). Doctors continue to guard the right to diagnose, regarding this as a medical prerogative based on their responsibility for the management of individual patients (Walby and Greenwell *et al.* 1994; Brown and Seddon 1996). Recognition of the different roles of doctors and nurses could lead to ambivalent feelings among some respondents about the benefits of claiming expertise in advanced bioscience.

> Nurses want to move away from medics, so we back away from biology and the handmaiden role. Biology shackles nursing to medicine and a subordinate role. [...] We can never equalise medics at their own game and medical models. They won't let you have a say on drugs. Challenging the doctors increases their fear – they reassert their dominance and right to control. Knowledge is power. (Comparator student, psychiatric hospital)

This extract accurately captures the perception of many nurses, who have been influenced by the 'new nursing', that advanced bioscience knowledge is closely associated with the 'medical model', and in turn with a hierarchical division of labour in which the nurse is subordinate to the doctor. From this standpoint, role changes that bring nurses more clearly into the bio-medical domain will erode their claim to a separate knowledge base and ultimately strengthen medical control. Commentators such as Walby and Greenwell *et al.* (1994) argue that lack of cohesion amongst nurses, with some resenting the establishment of an elite, is acting as a barrier to the advancement of nursing as a profession. Certainly our data suggest that professional divisions do constrain nurses' ability to apply advanced bioscience knowledge effectively.

Perhaps, as a way of minimising conflict, much communication about nurses' expanded knowledge took a coded or understated form. Thus, several nurses complained that their contribution to important patient management decisions was often not rewarded with due praise.

An old lady, vomiting and constipated, was assumed to be in obstruction. I found out she was on dig. [Digoxin] and I suggested measuring for 'dig tox' [digitalis toxicity] and the potassium. It was found up. The 'dig' was stopped. That meant no surgery. She went home. The constipation was long standing. That was quite a little victory, but it was pushed under the carpet. (Staff nurse, surgical unit)

In this extract, the metaphor of 'victory' suggests that conflict and turf battles continue to be central features of nurses' everyday experience of the hospital division of labour. However, it is apparent that nurses are becoming increasingly sophisticated observers of their own professional situation. Academic constructs such as the 'doctor–nurse game' (Stein 1967; Fairman 1992; Ryan 1996) now figure explicitly in nurse education and are beginning to enter nurses' own discourses.

It's everyone's knowledge. You play the doctor–nurse game. Make the doctor think he thought about it first. It's time consuming, day in, day out, bartering with people. Doctors dump routine onto nurses – a venous blood sample is bartered for a prescription [...] Doctors are no help with leg ulcers, a specialist nurse know best. Doctors hand this sort of thing over to nurses [...] I know more than the GP now. For example now, pain control in terminal illness – he (patient) couldn't swallow – I wanted a syringe driver instead of oral MST. The GP walked off. (District nurse)

If you barge in, it'll just blow everything up, so I say 'Can I ask your advice on this?' [...] You tell them what to do. The renin-angiotensin system. He [doctor] asked me and I told him. He said most surgeons wouldn't know as much as I did on that. I don't feel as if I'm infringing. It wouldn't get done otherwise. (Staff nurse, surgical unit)

In these and other extracts, respondents showed their awareness of the fragile and contestable status of claims to expertise that they might make: new patterns of inter-professional working had to be informally negotiated and might need to be adjusted according to circumstances and the parties involved.

Nurses reported that doctors were more likely to support nurse autonomy in 'borderline' territory, such as wound care:

Doctors will prescribe as asked, except for the cost. [...] They don't know much about wound care. Physicians are more receptive than surgeons. (Specialist nurse, ulcer clinic)

Similarly, in the CMHN study, doctors were prepared to cede control of medical practice at the margins, and were willing for nurses to monitor patients for the side effects of the medications they had prescribed. Four CMHNs (taking the students and controls together) had encountered resistance from medical practitioners, but seven had found that psychiatrists were supportive of their efforts to improve side effect monitoring. The remaining three CMHNs did not comment on this issue when they talked about constraints.

The potential of the nursing pharmacology course to impact on patient care was limited by the nurses' professional 'territory' and the resource constraints of the service. While some aspects of client monitoring were considerably improved, others showed little or no change, despite equal attention on the course. Although the CMHNs could monitor for side effects by weighing clients, taking blood pressures, and encouraging dental inspections, they were not authorised to organise ECGs. Authorisation of diagnostic tests of this kind remained firmly under medical control. Over the period of the study there was no change in the frequency of ECG recordings. Students spoke of the difficulties of implementing the course recommendation on cardiac monitoring for patients receiving high doses of anti-psychotic medication (BNF 2001).

> It's all very well suggesting that Joe Bloggs has an ECG but if the GP won't sign the thing, then *tough*. It's not done on the ward. If they've had a relapse and been on loads of medication, they come back from the ward, but if it's not done then, when there are no costs attached, what chance of you having it done once they're out? [...] But I've never known anybody have an ECG in my whole ten years of working at [name of hospital], and that's people who have been on anti-psychotics for 10 or 15 years, in huge doses. [...] We are only going to get frustrated in the end, because we think that someone should have an ECG, but the doctor won't request it. (CMHN, immediately post-course)

While this nurse was now aware of the cardiotoxic side effects of anti-psychotics, she felt powerless to change practice. The incongruence between the BNF guidelines highlighted on the course and the realities of practice led to feelings of frustration, with both the course and the limitations of nursing's professional role boundaries. Respondents felt that without managerial support, or a managerially driven audit, initiatives, such as regular monitoring, were unlikely to be sustained in the long term. Similar views have been expressed by nurses in other studies (Nolan *et al.* 1995; Francke *et al.* 1995; Dowling *et al.* 1996).

The burgeoning literature on iatrogenic neglect indicates that these instances of suboptimal care may not be untypical of routine practice (Royal College of General Practitioners 1985; Lindley *et al.* 1992; Zermansky 1996; Harris and Dajda 1996; Denneby *et al.* 1996; Cunningham *et al.* 1997; Stevens and Balon 1997; Rokstad and Straand 1997; Rochon and Gurwitz 1997; Roughead *et al.* 1998; Pirmohamed *et al.* 1998; Wallace and Solomon 1999; Gandhi *et al.* 2000; Pouyanne *et al.* 2000; Kohn *et al.* 2000). Accordingly, official reports, user groups and academics have called for an examination of practice in relation to medication management (Chapman 1991; Garvey *et al.* 1991; Department of Health and RCN 1994; Department of Health 1994; Wright and Parker 1998), and the introduction of national standards (NHS 2000).

Some of these problems may be emanating from medicine's professional monopoly on medication management. Extending the professional education and role boundaries of nursing may be one strategy to curtail the potential for iatrogenesis. However, this draws nurses into the sensitive area of checking doctors' practice: a task that few relish.

Policing the doctors

There is a growing view that doctors, nurses and support staff should work as team players, and that staff of all grades have an obligation to point out errors and report untoward events. For example, the recent Bristol Royal Infirmary Inquiry Report (Kennedy 2001) suggests that all staff have an obligation to report 'sentinel events', and recommends that this is made as easy as possible, with those coming forward being given immunity from disciplinary action. The advanced courses examined in this chapter equipped students to better monitor the side effects of prescribed medications. This meant that they might be placed in situations where they were required to check decisions already made by medical practitioners, and that they might in effect be seen to be policing medical prescribing. An example summarised from an academic diary illustrates the kinds of situations that could arise:

> A diploma student working as a staff nurse on a surgical ward recognised a serious drug interaction in a patient co-prescribed amiodarone and digoxin. An elderly male patient had been taking digoxin for several years, but after his operation for an inguinal hernia, he developed symptomatic cardiac arrhythmias. Without adjusting or monitoring the digoxin, the registrar initiated the prescription of amiodarone. This interaction was predictable from pharmacokinetic principles. Both the metabolic and the renal actions of amiodarone reduced the clearance of digoxin, which accumulated within a few days. The high concentration of digoxin caused nausea and vomiting, leading to dehydration (Smith 1991). Dehydration promoted thrombus formation (Tierney 1995), and the patient developed a popliteal embolus. The digoxin and amiodarone combined failed to control the patient's atrial fibrillation. Although randomised controlled trials indicate that the risk of stroke justifies the use of anticoagulants in patients with atrial fibrillation (Caro et al. 1993), anticoagulants were prescribed only after the advent of the popliteal embolus. The cause of the digitalis toxicity, vomiting and dehydration was recognised by the nurse. Only when alerted by the nurse did medical staff adjust the dose of digoxin. Had the nurse not intervened, coma and death could have followed. [Both the BNF (2001) and Stockley (1999) state that if amiodarone is co-prescribed with digitalis, the dose of digitalis should be halved. Why this was not done before the nurse intervened is not clear]

Medication monitoring might be said to be a task over which no single occupation exercises clear jurisdiction. From the standpoint of doctors, it is one of many concerns embedded in routine interactions with patients undertaken for multiple purposes, and it may not have great visibility. Many nurses will have been taught that medication monitoring is a nursing task, but lack the advanced knowledge required to develop a useful role in this area. The lack of a clear division of labour, and a clear allocation of responsibilities, means that this is an area where inter-professional conflict is a distinct possibility. CMHNs, who had completed the course and were putting their new knowledge to use by checking for drug interactions and side effects, often found themselves reviewing doctors' prior prescribing decisions. On occasion, this could mean nurses approaching doctors with requests to re-consider past decisions. In the following example, the nurse describes how she now had the 'confidence' to express her unhappiness with a long-standing therapeutic regime:

I am much more knowledgeable and I actually know what I am doing now, and I question what I am doing. That came out more than anything when I went to see about Mrs [name] She has been on Lorazepam 30 mg per day for 32 years*. She was on four different anti-depressants plus thyroxine. [...] Plus she was buying medications over the counter and drinking. She fell and fractured her femur, recovered and went back to [...] hospital, fell, re-fractured the same femur, and had a bone graft. She nearly died that time. Now she's back home and I'm visiting two or three times a week. [...] I do feel that now I have got more knowledge. I felt more confident to say to the doctor that I was not happy with the medication, and I wanted it reviewed, and we should be looking at a reduction. (CMHN, 6 months post-course) [*BNF (2001) dose for Lorazepam is up to 4 mg per day.]

Examples like this, taken together with the findings from earlier research (Rupp 1992; Miller 1995; Schneider *et al.* 1995; Bonfiglio *et al.* 1997), suggest that these nurses were sometimes acting as a 'second check' to doctor prescribers. However, this was not necessarily something that they welcomed. Although the nurses were prepared to intervene when absolutely necessary, they did not view this as their role. Furthermore, with additional insight into the complexities of medication management, nurses were more, not less, reluctant to undertake nurse prescribing. Students were not reassured by the North American literature, which reports the safety of nurse prescribing (Spitzer *et al.* 1974; US Office of Technology Assessment 1986). Rather, they expressed concern over the legal implications of nurse prescribing, and the possibility of role conflicts with doctors.

Nurse prescribing: 'I don't feel skilled enough'

Nurse prescribing is high on the current policy agenda. Both the *Crown Report* (Department of Health 1999), and the *Higher Level of Practice: Descriptors and Standards* (UKCC 1999) propose the widespread introduction of nurse prescribing. Implementation of *The NHS Plan* (NHS 2000) will entail fundamental changes in nursing roles, with nurses independently delivering complete episodes of care, including, for the majority of nurses, prescribing. However, by breaking the medical monopoly on prescribing, nurse prescribing may be viewed as both a challenge to medicine's hegemony and a cost-containment exercise (Department of Health 1989). There is little evidence that practising nurses have either been widely consulted or made an informed choice on the assumption of prescribing authority.

In evaluating our specialist course, we specifically sought respondents' views on nurse prescribing, at interview. It was suggested that a specialist course, targeted at the most common medications prescribed for mental illness would lay the foundations for nurse prescribing. However, increased sensitisation to the complexities and uncertainties in psychopharmacology made respondents more cautious about the additional responsibilities of prescribing. Similar concerns were expressed by nurse practitioners prescribing drugs for mental illness in the USA (Flenniken 1997). It is possible that the 'shame and blame' attached to medication errors may be deterring nurses from assuming greater responsibilities for medication management (Arndt 1994; Gladstone 1995). The majority (8/14, 6 students, 2 comparators) of our respondents were opposed to nurse prescribing, viewing the added responsibility with trepidation:

> I am not happy about nurse prescribing. Basically, I think it might be minor things at the moment, but I don't feel skilled enough to prescribe anything. [...] I don't think I have got the knowledge base to prescribe from scratch, to make a decision what to put somebody on. I don't know enough about general medicine, or the skills. At the end of the day, we are not doctors – I see that as a very different profession. I think we have got to be careful not to try and medicalise ourselves too much. (CMHN, care of older people 6 months post-course)

It should be noted that this response comes from a respondent who had made more effort than many to develop a medication-monitoring role. For example, she requested therapeutic drug monitoring for a patient taking phenytoin who appeared drowsy and, as a result of this intervention, prescribing of this drug was discontinued about six months later. But while this student saw monitoring as acceptable, prescribing was a step too far. Six of our respondents (five comparators and only one student) expressed some willingness to prescribe, and then only if they were offered further training to augment their knowledge gained by experience. The main reason cited in favour of nurse prescribing was convenience, particularly in semi-rural areas (for comparison, see Cooke and Standing 1995; Rufli 1996; Luker *et al.* 1997).

> It [prescribing] would be very advantageous in some respects. Say we go to a client's house and they're having side effects. You have to ring the doctor in [name of hospital] and ask to go ahead and give the client some procyclidine before you can do it. We carry procyclidine with us, but we have to go through the rigmarole of ringing somebody. Similarly, perhaps you get a call, usually on a Friday night; somebody's gone into a crisis. You go out, and again, it would be advantageous to people to be able to give something to ease their anxiety. But again, you have to go through the rigmarole of 'phoning the on-call GP or the doctor at [name of hospital] and getting it verified. [...] You have to get the OK before you can sort it out. Sometimes the client hasn't got a 'phone in the house and you've got to go looking for a 'phone and all that. (CMHN, comparator 6 months post-course)

Although most respondents were reluctant to prescribe, they were generally willing to adjust medication doses, on an 'as needed' basis. Under the proposals in the Crown Report (Department of Health 1989), CMHNs will be given authority to adjust the doses of their clients' medication within a range specified by the prescribing doctor. To some extent, this was seen as legitimising or consolidating existing practice, rather than the assumption of new responsibilities. Several respondents favoured this kind of approach:

> I think there are probably lots of issues around nurse prescribing which would need clearing up. [...] I wonder if rather than prescribing, it would be easier within dosage boundaries, say within a set range, and you can alter that accordingly. I can see that happening. I think in some ways it probably happens, in the sense that you go to visit someone, and find there are problems with the medication, and you go back to the consultant and say 'these are the problems, what do you think about the dose?' Then that will be done. In a sense it's you making the judgement, because it's you who has seen the person. At the end of the day, the consultant has authorised and signed, but it's you who decided to go back to him. (CMHN, immediately post-course)

Respondents were clear that dose titration depended on close liaison with prescribers (Rufli 1996). All but two of the respondents were willing to titrate dosages within a limited range:

> In a way we are doing this [titrating], but I wouldn't really call that nurse prescribing. [...] Because I know these people so well, I will ring the consultant and say that the client is going downhill again and ask the consultant to put him on Prozac instead of having a tricyclic, because that has never worked well with him, and the consultant is happy to do that. But I think it is because of the kind of client he is and the relationship I've got with him. (CMHN, 6 months post-course)

During the field observations dose titration was seen to operate. When a student found a client to be unduly stiff, a dose of anti-psychotic medication was withheld until problems had been checked with the consultant, who duly reduced the dose. Due to the close relationship with their clients, the CMHNs were aware of clients' preferences and idiosyncratic or hypersensitive reactions, which facilitated medication adjustment. This is particularly important for anti-psychotic medications where there is a wide variation in individuals' responses to any one drug. By equipping the nurses to monitor for interactions and side effects, the course facilitated dose titration. However, there was a perception among the students that, even with 33 taught hours, it was too limited in scope and duration to support nurse prescribing.

Increased status or survival?

Most respondents took the view that CPE was unlikely to improve their status or career prospects. Despite the view of the comparator quoted earlier that those completing advanced physiology courses were more interested in promotion than patient care, none of the respondents involved with CPE mentioned career advancement. Even where nurses were undertaking tasks that were previously the preserve of doctors, they were not expecting an increase in either pay or status:

> We're taking things off the doctors – IV's (intravenous infusions), defibrillation, venous bloods. This isn't an increase in status; neither is the qualification, diploma in nursing. (Sister, coronary care)

Within the routinised contexts of particular clinical settings, most aspects of the work proceeded as usual, with few changes in inter-personal relationships or personal power. Generally speaking, the respondents recognised that any role changes that followed course completion had to be negotiated within the framework of existing professional hierarchies. While increased bioscience knowledge might change the tone of relationships, it did nothing to modify the structural position of individual nurses in relation to their organisational superiors.

I'm far more knowledgeable about physiology, but I'm not more powerful. [...] Clinical competence keep jobs but this isn't an increase in status. Neither is the DN [Nursing Diploma]. (Staff nurse, surgical unit)

As the reference to 'jobs' in this extract implies, many nurses saw the completion of advanced courses as being more about safeguarding their position than advancing it. The two studies were completed at two points in the 1990s when the National Health Service (NHS) was affected by a series of organisational changes that were affecting the position of nursing staff. The development of NHS Trust management structures, the introduction of clinical directorates, and the growing concern with financial and quality management, often led to tensions between managers and professionals (e.g. Griffiths and Hughes 2000).

General managers had emerged as a powerful group within NHS Trusts and indeed many nurses had entered management to advance their careers. Several respondents expressed concerns about position in relation to managers and the managerial agenda for change.

Management hire and fire [...] Nursing models, they won't protect nurses in a job. Nurses hope to protect themselves by education. (Comparator CMHN, on generic course)

Only clinical input is keeping your job secure. Management [knowledge] will be less secure than clinical competence. In general areas there's going to be a handful of trained staff and carers will be doing all the work. Nurses are re-trenching in clinical competence – biology based. (Sister, surgical unit)

This last respondent succinctly expresses the fear shared by many others that in future a reduced proportion of qualified staff may find themselves working alongside a larger number of health care assistants (HCAs), trained via the National

Vocational Qualification (NVQ) route rather than diploma or degree courses. For these respondents, completing advanced physiology courses represented a way of enhancing professional competence, and reinforcing the difference between nurses and the new generation of support workers.

> NVQs' lack the knowledge. They don't know what they're doing. They'll do your job on half your salary. [...] Only technical, specialised knowledge is keeping our jobs. Nobody can replace you. (District nurse)

> NVQs lack biological knowledge. [...] Nursing jobs may be threatened if we move away from the physiological side of things. Devaluation of the nursing profession is a risk. (Staff nurse, EMI)

> Clinical competence keeps jobs. (Sister, cardiology)

CPE courses with a substantial bioscience content were seen as particularly relevant to this issue of clinical competence, presumably because it opened the way for nurses to make claims to a corpus of specialised knowledge that overlapped with that of the medical profession. Softer aspects of nursing's developing knowledge base, such as 'nursing models' were not seen to strengthen nurses' position to the same extent as biological knowledge.

> Nursing models won't protect nurses in a job. Nurses hope to protect themselves by education. (CMHN)

While – as we saw earlier – one subgroup of respondents expressed reservations about the medicalisation of nursing, another subgroup suggested that being a 'loving nurse' is no substitute for clinical competence.

> It's not good enough to say 'I don't know' to a relative. Basically, if a member of my family was being nursed, I'd hope the nurse would know about the body. You can't practice without it. It's all very well having a loving nurse, but if she doesn't know if the patient is blue to give cardiac massage, she's not much cop. (Staff nurse, A & E)

In many ways the worries and preoccupations of this group of nurses exemplify the dilemmas of nursing's professional project. If nurses embrace the approach of the 'new nursing' by distancing themselves from 'medical work' and emphasising holistic care, they risk a putative skills devaluation which weakens their labour market position *vis-à-vis* health care assistants.

However, if nurses seek to acquire advanced bioscience knowledge and accept a degree of medicalisation of nursing work, they once again fall under the shadow of the medical profession. Arguably, this illustrates the complexities that arise when a professional project is carried forward within an ecology of organisations already colonised by the established profession of medicine. The aspiring profession must content itself with a qualified acceptance, based on limited and uneven advances in areas which are not attractive to the dominant profession, and which results in considerable angst and ambivalence about the way forward.

Conclusion

This chapter has been partly about organisational constraints that limit the extent of role change following CPE, and partly about limits that nurses completing courses put on role change because of their perceptions of what is desirable.

Both cohorts of students applied their enhanced bioscience knowledge in areas such as increased vigilance for the side effects of medication. Generally, this was an area that accounted for little of doctors' time, and might be seen as unoccupied professional territory. The most significant barriers to this role expansion came from the nursing hierarchy and management, who were mostly unwilling to modify directorate or ward policies to accommodate such change. Some doctors were also unenthusiastic about nurses' involvement in these areas, but many respondents reported that they had negotiated an informal division of labour that allowed them a role in areas like medication monitoring. However, when coupled with pressures of time and resources, these factors served to curtail the extent of real change.

Moreover, the limited nature of change was also a reflection of respondents' limited aspirations. While all respondents said that they valued the courses they had completed, and almost all reported that they paid increased attention to medication monitoring, few wanted to go much further. There was little enthusiasm for a role that would involve systematic checking of doctors' prescribing, and a widespread view that they were not ready to move into the area of nurse prescribing. Respondents talked about their reasons for pursuing advanced courses more in terms of staying in a job rather than career advancement, and in this sense looked to their new qualifications as a means of maintaining the *status quo* rather than engineering fundamental role changes.

These findings raise the issue of the kind of educational provision that will be required if nurses are to move into the expanded roles foreshadowed in recent policy documents, such as *The NHS Plan* (NHS 2000). The Plan makes no explicit recommendations about the changes in nurse education that will be needed to allow 'at least 50%' of nurses to prescribe safely from 'an extended range of medicines' by 2004. The courses we have been considering were designed in response to the virtual absence of formal pharmacology content from many current pre-registration nurse education programmes, and were intended to enhance capability within present role structures rather than to prepare nurses to prescribe. However, they highlight the steep learning curve involved, and the lack of confidence that may hold nurses back. Longer, more intensive CPE courses may be part of the answer to these problems, as may an expansion of the pharmacology input in pre-registration education. However, organisational constraints of the kind discussed in this paper will also need to be addressed. If innovations such as nurse prescribing are to succeed, co-ordinated changes in policy and procedures in the clinical areas, and clear support from management and senior professionals must buttress CPE.

7 Creating a 'participatory caring context' on hospital wards

Davina Allen

Introduction

Sociological theories of the division of labour have been extensively employed to examine the boundaries between nursing work and other occupational groups, but there is rather less empirical research that has used this perspective to analyse the interface between nurses and unwaged 'lay' health workers, that is patients and their families and significant others (*pace* Strauss *et al.* 1985; Hughes 1984; Rosenthal *et al.* 1980).[9] This gap in the literature reflects the fact that it is only relatively recently that the healthcare work of lay people is beginning to be recognised and acknowledged. For many years, both public policy and academic theorising in this area were underpinned by a view of the lay–professional interface that assumed a passive role for patients and their families. Like other occupational divisions of labour, however, the lay–professional interface is historically bounded and currently undergoing processes of change. Both within nursing and the wider healthcare context efforts are currently being made to move towards a new model of professionalism (and hence, patienthood) (e.g. Stacey 1992; Witz 1994; Davies 1995) which is based on engagement, partnership and greater user control. As a consequence, this key caring division of labour is coming under increased scrutiny. In this chapter I employ a division of labour perspective to explore how the lay–professional interface was negotiated on two acute hospital wards in a large University teaching hospital in the United Kingdom (UK). Both wards espoused participatory models of practice but experienced different degrees of success in accomplishing their aims. The reasons for this variance are explored. Contrary to much of the professional literature which tends to emphasise the need for practitioners to change the nature of their relationship with service users, I suggest that, to a considerable extent, the roots of participatory practice may be found in features of the work setting.

Nurses, patients and their friends and family: changing boundaries, changing relationships

From 'sick role' to service consumer

Traditionally, the nurse–patient relationship was founded on an 'acute-care' model like that depicted by Parsons (1951) in his writings on the sick role. Taking their cues from the medical profession, which they sought to emulate (Rafferty 1996), nurse–patient relationships were characterised by affective neutrality, an emphasis on physical care, and an asymmetry of knowledge and patient passivity (Armstrong 1983). Once a person was admitted to a hospital, family involvement in the care of their kin was extremely limited and contact tightly restricted. Outside of designated visiting times, access to hospital wards was denied to all but 'inmates' (Goffman 1961) and staff.

In more recent years, however, this model of care has given way to a more holistic approach, based on a partnership between the nurse, patient and their significant others. In parallel with a wider 'democratic impulse' which has led to the questioning of hierarchical relationships in late modern cultures (Bury 2001), attempts have been made within nursing to equalise the imbalance of power that has traditionally characterised the lay–professional interface and to move away from models of care founded on passivity towards more active models based on shared decision-making and greater user control. Emphasis is given to the need to involve service users in the assessment, planning, provision (Ross 1987) and evaluation (Hefferin 1979; Hames and Stirling 1987) of care. Professional ideologies also underline the need for nurses to understand the subjective experience of the patient and their families and to use this knowledge to plan jointly packages of care centred on individual needs. Evidence of these trends is revealed in the burgeoning literature on patient empowerment (Gilbert 1995; Elliott and Turrell 1996), patient participation (Ashworth *et al.* 1992; Biley 1992; Jewell 1994), user involvement, family care, collaborative care (Waterworth and Luker 1990) and partnership working (Wade 1995).

Radical critiques of the professions

The impetus for the emergence of participatory models of practice within nursing came from multiple sources. One important influence was the sociological critiques of the professions that emerged during the 1960s and 1970s. Whereas earlier approaches to the study of the professions, such as that of Parsons (1951), regarded the power imbalance between professionals and the lay public to be a necessary consequence of their differential expertise, others were more critical. Writers such as Johnson (1967), Larson (1977) and Freidson (1970a,b) argued that social scientific scholarship had naively accepted the rhetoric and ideology of the established professions and reproduced this in their theories. They argued that, far from reflecting the essential nature of the lay–professional interface, the structural inequalities that characterised the professional–patient relationship were produced by the professions themselves in order to safeguard their power and justify their occupational privileges. Rather than serving disembodied social needs, professions imposed their own definitions of needs onto clients and were therefore a vehicle of social control. Proponents of the radical view maintained that the increased dominance of the medical profession was having an iatrogenic effect on society, de-skilling lay people and taking away their ability to care for themselves or deal with ordinary troubles and hardships (Illich 1976). It was also considered to be the cause of many of the perceived inadequacies of healthcare systems of this time (Freidson 1970a).

Consumerism

In the UK, evidence of the impact of these critiques may be found, *inter alia*, in the strong consumerist thread in recent public policy. In the healthcare context, for example, these trends were first evident in the Griffiths Report (Department of Health and Social Security 1983) which criticised health services for being more concerned with the needs of providers than with users. The ensuing period has seen the progressive reconstruction of the public from passive recipients of health-care into knowledgeable consumers and service users. Initially, new consumerism in healthcare was couched in terms of the language of the market. The current Labour government prefers to talk in terms of partnership and collaboration, but this is a change in presentation rather than substance. Indeed, the rhetoric of patient-centred care has become a vehicle for driving through changes to service organisation – such as role-realignment, new systems of clinical governance and multi-skilling – which would have been much more difficult to effect deploying new right discourses of efficiency.

The radical critiques of the professions provided the catalyst for a host of empirical studies concerned with issues related to the professional–patient relationship. In particular, attention focused on communication and the failure of the medical profession to provide patients and their families with information about their condition and treatment (Roth 1963; Glaser and Strauss 1965, 1968; Quint 1972; McIntosh 1977). This was a prominent theme in the ensuing consumerist policy trends: there is now an expectation that patients and families will be informed fully about their illness and enabled to participate in decisions about their treatment. This has been given added impetus by the hugely increased availability of information about illness from a number of sources.

> Where once the bio-medical paradigm held sway (and where doctors jealously guarded its secrets), now lay people have access to an increasing range of information and ideas about the origins, course and outcomes of illness and its treatment. (Bury 2001: 268)

Self-care

Although much of the consumerist rhetoric centres on service user rights, it is also clear that policy makers believe that service users have responsibilities. Contemporary healthcare systems emphasise the importance of self-management and independence and individual responsibility for health and wellness.

This is evident in recent government policies focused on health improvement. One of the dangers of such an approach, however, is that the behaviourist assumptions that underpin it obscure the links between material conditions and health. Studies have consistently indicated that an individual's pattern of health and well-being is inextricably linked to their socio-economic circumstances (Department of Health and Social Security 1980; Acheson 1998) and that whilst material inequalities persist, healthcare consumers do not have the same freedom to make choices about their healthcare behaviours.

Changing patterns of illness

This re-fashioning of the lay–professional interface has not been wholly ideologically driven. It has also been precipitated by demographic changes and the shift from the centrality of acute illness – on which the orthodox model of the professional–client relationship was founded – to the predominance of chronic illness and degenerative conditions that require continuing care. The management of chronic conditions is often complex, requiring medications, special diets, exercise regimes and regular monitoring. Sufferers develop particular kinds of skills and knowledge derived from their lived experience of their condition, knowledge that is frequently superior to that of health professionals (MacIntyre and Oldman 1977). In recent years, there has been a burgeoning of support groups focused on a specific disease or condition that can be an important source of practical help and emotional support for sufferers and their families. In many instances where medical interventions are limited or unacceptable then sufferers are adding complementary and alternative therapies to their repertoire of health treatments.

Professionalisation processes

Given that the new consumerism in healthcare represents an attempt to curtail professional power, it is somewhat ironic that a further driver of the democratic impulse within nursing has been the professionalising aspirations of the nursing leadership. Although at one level these trends reflect an attempt to improve the quality of care patients receive, they also have to be understood in terms of nursing's aspirations to professional status. The new models of patienthood evident in healthcare more generally have become bound up with theories of nursing practice in order to provide a warrant for nursing's jurisdictional claims. The nursing function has been reconstructed in terms of a close therapeutic relationship between nurse and patients. It is through the formation of a unique 'healing association' that nurses are said to promote healing and this, it is argued, is nurses' unique contribution to healthcare and the basis for its occupational niche. Moreover, alignment with the patient and their family also legitimates the empowerment of nurses *vis-à-vis* doctors.

> If the patient is to enjoy freedom of choice and the nurse is to be the agent of this choice, then the nurse must also be empowered and have the freedom to make decisions as an autonomous practitioner. (Trnobranski 1994: 734)

Participatory care in nursing: service consumers and 'reluctant collaborators'

At the heart of consumerist health policies is a very particular model of the patient: the middle class healthcare user who has access to modern information technology and wishes to be an active and knowledgeable participant in decisions about their care and treatment. As we have seen, within the nursing context, these themes have also been overlaid with theories of caring.

There is, however, a growing body of evidence that indicates that at least certain sections of the general public are rather more equivocal about this new version of patienthood. In his study of participation in day surgery patients, Avis (1994) concludes that most of his research respondents subscribed to what might best be described as a mechanic's model of patienthood: they wanted their healthcare problems 'fixed' by experts but no further engagement with the process. Such an orientation is perhaps understandable in the day surgery context where contact with health professionals is inevitably brief, yet there is evidence to suggest that patients in different settings also want rather less engagement with the caring process than these new models of patienthood imply. In a rare study of therapeutic nursing, Ersser (1997) found that neither patients nor nurses referred to the therapeutic effects of the nurse–patient relationship. Caress' (1997) study of renal patients also reveals that after years of self-management patients did not feel they had the necessary knowledge to be active participants in decision-making about their care. An observational study of the lay–professional interface in a District General Hospital undertaken by the author (Allen 2001a) revealed that whereas patients were content to undertake discrete self-care tasks, such as measuring their own fluid balance, they were rather less enthusiastic about being involved in the planning of their care. In this instance, it was suggested that patient participation was driven principally by the desire to help overworked nursing staff, rather than any overriding desire to be an active patient. These findings echo Darbyshire's (1994) study of parental participation on paediatric wards.

This evidence has led some critics to suggest that the enthusiasm with which nurses have embraced participation in the clinical setting has led them to ignore its dynamic nature. 'Participation' is a complex concept covering a range of activities and different levels of involvement. As Salvage (1992) points out, acutely ill patients' predominant concerns are likely to be freedom from pain and discomfort rather than the establishment of a close caring association with their nurse. Certain nursing procedures involve crossing important social and personal boundaries, which may actually be made more manageable through the adoption of a detached stance (Avis 1994; Lawler 1991). Furthermore, lay people may wish for more power to make choices, participate in their care and assert their personal identities, but be very cautious about assuming responsibility for treatment decisions (Coyle 1999). As Dingwall (1996) has observed, it is relatively easy to obtain information about an illness or condition but much more difficult to know what it means. It is likely that lay people will always look to more knowledgeable 'intermediaries' to interpret the evidence and apply it to their particular case.

Weather-god or meterorologist, the professional is our means of reducing uncertainty about important things we cannot easily or economically verify for ourselves. (Dingwall 1996: 10)

Patients' ability and willingness to participate in their care is not fixed, moreover. It varies according to their state of health, the possession of knowledge about the issue at hand and the constraints of the healthcare setting (Biley 1992). There is, therefore, a real danger that the uncritical acceptance of the rhetoric of participation by nurses can lead to the imposition of a new version of patienthood which is equally as constraining as the orthodox sick role model.

Yet, while there is a clear need for a reflective approach to participation which avoids its imposition on 'reluctant collaborators' (Waterworth and Luker 1990), there is a growing body of evidence which indicates that, at the very least, the general public has a strong requirement that they should be treated as individuals (Baker and Lyne 1996; Ersser 1997; Coyle 1999). In a recent interview study of people who had experienced problems with the health service, Coyle (1999) found that 40 out of 41 respondents produced accounts that showed that untoward experiences were described in terms of how they undermined individual identity. These included perceptions of being: dehumanised, objectified, stereotyped, disempowered and devalued. Coyle deploys the notion of 'personal identity threat' to describe her findings. Her exposition points to the importance that people attached to attention being paid to their feelings and having their unique knowledge recognised. Dissatisfaction was expressed with standardised production-line style care and not being treated as an individual (see also, Attree 2001). There are clear similarities here with Allan's (2001) ethnographic study of a fertility clinic, which highlights the importance of 'emotional awareness'. This refers to 'a level of emotional support, which was not intense and did not involve emotional intimacy or closeness but where patients were aware of nurses' concern' (Allan 2001: 53).[10]

These findings indicate that whilst patients' ability and willingness to participate in their care may be highly variable, there appears to be a level of agreement that it should not undermine patients' sense of self. This still requires changes to the lay–professional interface and a reconsideration of how services are organised and delivered but it falls short of the more extreme versions of the active patient or 'healing association' which would lead to the imposition of a new version of patienthood on those who do not desire it. In a sense it provides the base-line participatory caring context against which the lay–professional interface can be mutually constituted on a case by case basis (Purkis 1996) and levels of participation negotiated and emotions engaged or disengaged according to the purposes at hand.

In the second part of this chapter I report on research undertaken on two wards both of which aspired to participatory models of care. Whilst a 'base-line' of participatory practice – of the kind described by Coyle (1999) and Allan (2001) – had been achieved in one setting, success in the other was partial. My aim is to examine the differences in the two settings in order to explain this variance.

The study

My initial interest in studying the lay–professional interface was stimulated by doctoral research into nurses' management of their work boundaries on a surgical ward and a medical ward in a large district general hospital (Allen 2001a, see also Chapter 2, this volume). This study revealed that although patients were more involved in self-care activities, lay–professional role relationships remained rooted in the traditional asymmetries of power characteristic of the Parsonian sick role. Because the lay–professional interface was an unanticipated theme in the original research I was unable to talk to patients about their participation in care. Ethical approval had not been obtained and resource restraints would not have allowed it. I was sufficiently excited by the original findings, however, to undertake further in-depth research.

The research was undertaken over a 4-month period in a large UK University teaching hospital. Two wards – surgery and medicine – were studied for 2 months each. The aim of the research was to explore how the lay–professional interface was negotiated in the acute setting, focusing on the healthcare work of patients and family carers and/or significant others (Allen 2000a,b, see also Chapter 8, this volume).

Ethical approval for the study was secured from the local research ethics committee. Written consent was obtained from all patients and their families who participated in the study, after they had been given time to consider fully whether they wanted to be involved or not. Access to the service setting was negotiated through the Director of Nursing in the first instance and thereafter through the medical and surgical directorate managers. I gave short presentations to ward staff in both settings in order to explain the purposes of the study and give them the opportunity to ask any questions or raise any concerns.

The wards were arranged each side of a central corridor and accommodated 19 patients on each side. In each case I was based on the north side. My research role ranged from observer to participant. Because much of what I was interested in was likely to take place 'behind the screens' (Lawler 1991) I negotiated an active participant–observer role. An honorary contract was agreed with the Trust that permitted me to work in the capacity of an auxiliary or health care assistant. Field observations were recorded in a spiral-bound shorthand notebook. My preference is to record a behaviourist record of what I see, rather than an interpretation of the meaning of a particular event. So, for example, if I witness a disagreement I will attempt to record the unfolding dialogue, rather than recording that 'X had a disagreement with Y'.

The observational material were supplemented by tape-recorded interviews with ward staff. Eleven staff nurses were interviewed on the surgical ward and four auxiliaries and nine qualified nurses on the medical ward. At the time of the study there were no auxiliaries/HCAs on the north side of the surgical ward. In addition extended non-tape-recorded conversations were carried out with a sample of patients and their carers. Thirteen patients and five carers were interviewed on the surgical ward and eleven patients and six carers were interviewed on the medical ward. For the most part these took place by the bedside, or occasionally in the day room. As far as possible these conversations were recorded contemporaneously. Interviews lasted between 30 minutes and one hour.

Theoretical framework

The research was informed by interactionist theories of the division of labour (Strauss *et al.* 1982a,b, 1985; Hughes

1984) in which care was defined as 'work'. Following Hughes, I was interested in the technical division of labour – that is the allocation of work between 'workers' at this interface – and the moral division of labour – that is the lay–professional role relationship: status, power and expertise (see also Chapter 1, this volume). The close linkage of these concepts is evident in standard definitions of participation found in the literature (e.g. Brownlea 1987). For example, increasing patient participation in the technical aspects of their care is one mechanism for effecting user empowerment by increasing control and independence, and this has been a key component of the movement towards greater patient participation in nursing. Yet, this link is by no means automatic. Patient involvement in the physical aspects of their care does not always bring about modifications to their role relationship with nurses and as we have seen, although most are agreed about the changes to the moral division of labour in healthcare maybe necessary, there is less agreement over changes to the technical division of labour. For this reason, following Hughes I prefer to keep the moral and technical divisions of labour conceptually distinct (Allen 2000a). I approached the fieldwork with the following questions: (i) what types of work does the provision of healthcare entail, (ii) who does that work, (iii) how is the work negotiated between those involved in the caring division of labour and (iv) what effect does the context in which care is given have on all of the above? Analysis was facilitated by the use of *FolioViews Information Production Kit 3.1*. Data were coded iteratively according to the analytic themes arising from the field and the study's guiding theoretical framework.

Creating a participatory caring context: the surgical ward

I began my fieldwork on the surgical ward and was immediately struck by its overall atmosphere. Collectively the staff had created what I have called a 'participatory caring context' (Allen 2000a). Patients and their families described them as 'warm', 'friendly' and 'approachable'.

They're all very approachable. (Fieldnotes – Relative)

> The nurses on here are wonderful though. Each time I've been on they've been great: you can ask them anything. It's very relaxed. Not like years ago when it was the stiff collar you know. (Fieldnotes – Patient)

> [T]he patients are more relaxed, they come up to the desk, you know you have a chat, they ask questions at the desk and the relatives as well. (Interview – Staff nurse)

So how did the staff achieve this warmth? At the time this was something one simply felt from being there, but further analysis and reflection suggest it had a number of constituent elements. These were: a culture of openness, a people-orientation and a focus on the individual.

A culture of openness

One component of the participatory caring context was the ward's culture of openness. The visiting policy permitted family members to visit at any time. Brooking (1989) has suggested that familiarity with the ward makes participation of family carers more likely. Moreover, ward activities are not hidden away and secretive. One nurse also indicated that because visiting was spread throughout the day, the nurses had more opportunity to spend time with people since they were not having to deal with everybody simultaneously. Nurses appeared to have good relationships with family members; they spoke to them at length, both face-to-face on the ward and on the telephone updating them on their loved ones' progress. They also worked hard to maintain patients' contact with the outside world and keep channels of communication open. Access was granted to the ward telephone and nurses relayed messages to and from bed-bound patients.

> The phone rings and staff nurse answers it.
> *Staff nurse*: Hello [surgical ward] staff nurse speaking.
> [*Pause*]
> OK would you like me to see if there's any message for you?
> [*Staff nurse goes off into the cubicle*]
> *Staff nurse*: He says just to tell you he's coming on fine.
> [*Pause*]
> He was in last night. (Fieldnotes)

The phone rang.

Staff nurse: Hello [surgical ward] nurse James speaking.
[*Pause*]
Staff nurse: Hi. It's Jenny speaking.
[*Pause*]
What had she had done when you last called?
[*Pause*]
Yes. Well she had that done yesterday and she had a bit of pain last night but she's OK now. Do you have a message you'd like me to pass on?
[*Pause*]
By all means. No problem.
[*Pause*]
By all means. That's not a problem at all. (Fieldnotes)

This culture of openness also extended to communication and information giving on the ward. Nurses were very proactive in providing information to patients and their families and in encouraging them to ask questions. The nursing staff had developed information leaflets for the main conditions suffered by patients admitted to the ward, which they gave to people on admission.

They say anything you want to know don't leave it to yourself – ask and I do and most of the time they have the right answers. (Fieldnotes – Patient)

[T]hey are so free with their information here. When you ask it's never too much trouble to take time to explain it. They don't just say to you 'Oh that's nothing. That's just for his stomach'. They explain – 'Well you know it's for the acid in his stomach' or 'It's to stop the pain'. Because there are two different tablets. One is for the pain in his stomach, the other is for the acid in his stomach and they take time to explain that bit to you. (Fieldnotes – Relative)

They're very helpful – the nurses. If you ask them a question, they'll tell you. They're not holding anything back. (Fieldnotes – Patient)

I think we feel less intimidated. If there are things to say then we will tell people – you know. We don't hold on to information as much like a lot of people do. (Interview – Staff nurse)

Nurses responded to queries and requests openly and fully and demonstrated a respect for the knowledge and contribution of patients and their families. This was in marked contrast to the defensive stance I have observed elsewhere (Allen 2000a, 2001a).

People-orientation

Coyle (1999) notes that one way in which encounters with health service providers can threaten self-identity is by the failure of health professionals to adhere to the normal rules of social interaction. Drawing on the work of Strauss *et al.* (1982b), Garfinkel (1967) and Goffman (1959, 1963, 1971), Coyle points out that normal social interaction is governed by taken-for-granted rules. If these rules are obeyed they remain invisible, but when they are broken the interactant will be perceived as rude or inappropriate. As a number of observers have pointed out (Strauss *et al.* 1982b; Menzies 1963; Latimer 2000; Allan 2001), the social organisation of medical work can lead health providers to break these taken-for-granted rules. For example, Allan (2001) describes an incident in which a clinic nurse, having spent five minutes arranging an appointment with an extremely anxious patient, turned her back on her to sort out some notes, and ignored the woman until she eventually withdrew from the clinic.

For the most part, the nurses on the surgical ward displayed a strong orientation to the maintenance of normal rules of social interaction. Nurses always introduced themselves when they were meeting with patients and their families for the first time, and identified themselves personally when answering the telephone. Relatives were always acknowledged on the ward and the nurses displayed genuine interest in their well being. This could range from a simple acknowledgement of their co-presence to a more empathetic concern with their welfare. There are clear resonances here with the two aspects of 'emotional awareness' – described by the participants in Allan's (2001) study: 'knowing what I am going through' and 'being there in the background'.

> A relative is walking down the ward corridor
> *Student nurse*: OK?
> *Relative*: Yes – fine.   (Fieldnotes)

> A relative of the patient in the cubicle who is dying is going back into the room. He has just made himself a drink. Cindy [staff nurse] is writing in some notes at the nurses' station. As the relative walks past she asks:
> *Staff nurse*: All right?

Rel: [*Quietly*] Yes thanks.   (Fieldnotes)

As we are talking, two of Dora's relatives emerge from the cubicle. I had seen them talking to the consultant earlier who had told them that Dora's prognosis was not good and that she was very poorly. As they emerge from the cubicle Paula [staff nurse] breaks off our conversation.

Staff nurse: Are you OK?

Female relative: Yes. [*She doesn't sound so sure*]. She's not very well.

Staff nurse: Her chest isn't very good.

Female relative: No. There's nothing more they can do.

Staff nurse: Have you spoken to Mr [name]?

Female relative: Yes. [*Begins to leave the ward – visibly distressed*].

Staff nurse: You take care now.   (Fieldnotes)

This people-orientation was also evident in nurses' interactions with the patients. I frequently observed the nurses informing the patients of their work plans. This meant patients were not left in a state of uncertainty wondering when, for example, the nurse was coming to change their dressing or assist them in the bathroom, and it also gave patients more control over their use of time. Studies have shown that negotiation over the 'passage of time' is an important element of the moral division of labour between lay people and health professionals (see also Chapter 2, this volume). Roth (1963) has highlighted the importance of establishing a timetable in reducing uncertainty over the recovery trajectory for people suffering from TB.

I was sitting at the nurses' station looking through some patient case notes. Sharon [staff nurse] came to the trolley outside the cubicles and started putting on a plastic apron. Both the patients in the cubicles have MRSA infections. Sharon popped her head round Peter's door.

Staff Nurse: I won't be a minute then I'll be in. I'm just going to sort out this lady.   (Fieldnotes)

A focus on individuals

A further contributor to the participatory caring context on the surgical ward was nurses' strong sense of ownership and responsibility for their patients. They went to considerable lengths to maintain continuity of care and knew patients and their families well.[11] On one occasion I observed nurses resisting the transfer of an 'outlier medical patient'[12] to another ward because he would not know anyone, even though he was 'blocking' a valuable 'surgical bed'.

> When Jane [staff nurse] came off the phone she announced: They're moving Boris to Friends Ward!
>
> *DA*: When?
>
> *Staff nurse*: Today? It seems silly to move him just for a few days. He knows everyone here. He won't know anyone there. But then he is blocking a vascular bed. (Fieldnotes)

A further expression of the surgical nurses' focus on individuals was their willingness to work flexibly to accommodate patient needs and preferences whilst recognising the constraints of certain hospital and ward routines (see also Chapter 2, this volume).

> I can't get over how relaxed and laid back it is on here. How can they do that? There's no pressure to do things at a certain time. They always ask if you want to do something and if you don't then you can do it later. (Fieldnotes – Relative)

> [W]e're not very fussy sort of in the way we don't make beds at a strict time, we don't get them all out of bed. [...] we've altered our style so much that people think we're messy and sloppy. But some of it is that we don't all do beds, some of it is not totally our fault but then we will let patients guide their own events. We don't slap them all in the bath. [...] we do let them decide – I'll say you know 'Well do you want it later or'. (Interview – Staff nurse)

The nurses also demonstrated a readiness to bend the rules rather than sticking slavishly to protocol in order to accommodate individual needs and were respectful of the patient's perspective and their knowledge of their condition.

> [W]e sometimes get patients with Berger's disease and they've got like black finger-tips and that and they absolutely hate you doing their dressings and sometimes will point blank refuse 'No – I'll do my own dressing'. So say they'll do their own dressing. So probably at home say – they will do things – their own dressings anyway. So what we tend to do with them is: we go in with them, make sure they wash their hands and you know just use the correct technique. It may not be aseptic but it will be clinically clean. You know – so that's one way I suppose of overcoming problems. It's just to work with the patient and as I say be flexible in the end. You know we can't be rigid. (Interview – Staff nurse)

> Staff nurse [Sharon] is doing the blood sugars before breakfast. She goes to the new patient [*admitted from County Hospital with constipation*].

Staff nurse: I just want to do your BM. Actually do you want to do this because you do it at home don't you?

Patient: Yes.

[*The patient does his own BM. Sharon reads the result*]

Staff nurse: Did you start off with strips and then go on to a machine?

Patient: That's right yes. (Fieldnotes)

Meehan (1981) argues that one way in which the lay–professional boundary is maintained in face-to-face encounters in medical settings is through the use of jargon. Medical jargon provides an efficient way of communicating shared knowledge and provides a common sense of identity for health professionals. For the lay person, however, the use of technical language can have a negative effect, precluding understanding. Moreover, the lay person by definition does not have access to the knowledge to which the jargon refers. My findings echo those of Pilnick (1998), however, who observes that patients and carers often use technical terms, and that health professionals appear to accept that patients have access to such knowledge. On the surgical ward, too, patients and their family frequently used medical terminology with no evidence of mitigators or qualifiers that would suggest that they were not legitimate users of such language.

Staff nurse: What's that tablet that we didn't get for you? Have you taken that?

Patient: Frusemide?

Staff nurse: Yes

Patient: Yes. I'm due some more tonight. (Fieldnotes)

We moved to Donald Green's bed. The student nurse retrieves the drug kardex and studies it. Once again she and the staff nurses discuss the tablets. Staff nurse is looking something up in the BNF. In the meantime the student has located some tablets in the trolley and begins to push them out of the bubble pack into the gallipot. The patient is looking at her and nodding.

Patient: That's right.

Student nurse: Donald! Have you had your Cisapride?

Patient: Yes I have it in the morning and the evening.

Student writes in 'self' in the drugs kardex against the drugs that Donald is administering himself. (Fieldnotes)

Care plans

Care plans are a key symbol of models of participatory practice in the nursing context. They are an indicator of nurses' unique holistic caring approach and in more recent years they have become a vehicle for nurse–patient partnerships (Jewell 1994). Neophyte nurses are exhorted to negotiate individually tailored plans of care in collaboration with the patient.

In one respect the nursing care plans on the surgical ward were an important marker of their caring philosophy. The ward nurses had adopted a new model of care planning, based on Orem's model of nursing (1995), which was different from that used elsewhere in the hospital. Care plans were written in the form of a contract between nurse and patient, as in the following anonymised example.

Robert Hart – diabetic care plan

Robert will:

1. Inform staff if feeling faint, flushed, dizzy, confused, nauseous.
2. Eat a reduced (sugar free) diet.
3. Learn to monitor his own blood sugars.

Nurses will:

1. Administer medication as prescribed.
2. Take and record blood sugar levels 4–6 hourly or pre-meal.
3. Refer to diabetic nurses.
4. Refer to dietician.
5. Encourage a sugar free diet.   (Document)

Yet, although the care plans created the impression of being individually negotiated, they were rarely agreed in this way. In fact, many of the care plans for routinely encountered conditions were standardised and available on pre-prepared plans. Even when care plans were tailored to individual patients they were not written with them. Apparently, when the new care planning system was introduced the nurses repeatedly found that patients had no interest in making such a contribution.

> We got quite disheartened by the amount of patients that didn't want to be involved – 'No you're the nurse you tell me what you are going to do'. I mean they do take on this sick role – there's very few that want to be involved. (Interview – Staff nurse)

This nurses' observations were confirmed over the course of the fieldwork. Although care plans were left at the end of the patients' beds, the patients rarely consulted them. The few patients who had looked at them talked about it in rather conspiratorial terms, such as 'having a sneaky look' or a 'peek', indicating that they did not regard themselves as legitimate readers of this document. Although the nurses were disappointed that patients did not want further involvement in their care planning, with the passage of time, they had concluded that formal participatory processes, such as care planning, were less important than the overall approach to care.

> I know we don't use, even the documentation now properly. [...] But if they're not doing it right it's not the end of the world. The main thing is your communication skills – in assessing the patient – and then you should be thinking forward any way I think. [...] I think it's just changing your views as to how you assess the patient I think. (Interview – Staff nurse)

> I mean half the time I do wonder what we're doing in terms of doing Orem correctly anyway. But I think the core point is to try and be more aware and try and get everyone geared up to the fact that we should be getting patients more involved in their care. We should respect what they want. (Interview – Staff nurse)

The nurses still valued the care plans – on a number of occasions staff referred proudly to their 'beautiful care plans' – but their importance lay in their value as a symbol of the ward philosophy rather than as a reflection of their actual practice.

Taken together then, these elements constituted the participatory caring context so evident on the surgical ward. It provided the backdrop against which negotiation of the lay–professional interface could take place on an individual basis.

Discussion

By underlining the importance of the context of care I have taken a rather different approach from that which dominates the nursing literature where writing on changing nurse–patient relationship stresses the importance of the practitioner's skills (Malin and Teasdale 1991; Elliott and Turrell 1996). For example, Elliott and Turrell (1996) present the contradictions of new models of patienthood in terms of the 'dilemmas for the empowering nurse' and recommend clinical supervision as a mechanism for managing these tensions. Whilst not denying the importance of individual nurses' interpersonal skills, I suggest that more attention needs to be given to effects of the environment on supporting participatory practice (also see, Davis 1980). It is true that social actors have a good sense of the 'role formats' (Strong 1979) or interactional 'frame' (Goffman 1974) available to lay people and professionals in healthcare settings, but whilst these stocks of knowledge broadly shape patterns of interaction, they do not provide clear scripts for action, and in each situation these roles have to be negotiated anew.

In hospital settings, much professional–client interaction takes place under conditions of high visibility (Davis 1980). A number of participant observers have highlighted that one of the ways in which the local interactional rules can be discerned in public settings such as hospital wards, is by observing patterns of interaction and behaviour. For example, in her account of being a parent on a paediatric ward, Webb (1977) describes how she learnt to be a 'good mother'. Webb suggests that there was no direct socialisation as such, rather parents had to learn from observation of others and through discussion with other mothers away from the ward. Webb notes that it seemed vital to learn accepted practices; making a mistake could be a humiliating process and the power of staff to enforce such negative sanctions made for a passive parent population. By creating a participatory caring context, the surgical ward nurses were able to provide an environment that was warm and supportive, and which encouraged those patients and families who wanted it to negotiate an active role for themselves, without forcing it upon those who did not.

In the second part of this chapter I am going to consider the medical ward, where staff had also embraced participatory philosophies of care, but had been rather less successful in realising their aspirations. During the course of the exposition I will compare key features of the organisation of work in each setting and begin to suggest certain factors that appear to inhibit or facilitate the creation of a participatory caring context.

Barriers to the creation of a participatory caring context: the medical ward

> Our aim is always to act professionally, but to also ensure that the ward atmosphere is warm and friendly, which we believe encourages more of a partnership between patients, their relatives or carers. (Document)

In many respects, the medical ward's mission statement encapsulates much of what had been achieved on the surgical ward, yet in the former setting these aspirations had been only partially realised. At one level, there were certain similarities between the two locales. An open visiting policy was in place and I observed staff facilitating communication between patients and their families. The nurses also recognised the importance of lay knowledge and had made some effort to integrate this into their practice and in face-to-face encounters (but, see also Chapter 8, this volume). Moreover, as with the surgical ward, staff generally upheld the taken-for-granted rules of social interaction. There were, however, many others aspects of the work organisation that undermined their aspirations for practice.

Openness?

Openness was mitigated by a number of factors. For example, owing to workload considerations, the ward operated a policy of restricting telephone inquiries to one family member who was expected to liase with other relatives. I also observed occasions when staff refused or were unable to disclose information. This contrasted markedly with the extended conversations I observed on the surgical ward. Moreover, unlike the surgical ward where nurses were able to provide service users with the information they needed, I frequently observed medical ward nurses referring such requests onto medical staff.

> Meanwhile the phone rings and I answer it.
> *Caller:* Could you tell me how [name] is?

DA: Who's calling?

Caller: It's his ex-wife – I'm calling on behalf of his son and daughter.

DA: If you'd like to hold the line I'll get the nurse who is looking after him.

[*I showed the name of the patient I'd written down to Gillian*]

Gillian: [*Starts to look through her scrap of paper*] I don't know him. He's not one of mine. He's in the nine bedder. [*Picks up phone*] Hello. [Pause] Who's calling?

[*Pause*]

I'm sorry I can't give out information over the phone. All I can say is that he is comfortable. You'll have to come in and see the doctors. He's not just come in today has he? He's been in a few days. He only came in with chest pain – that's all. Well not all – he came in with chest pain. [*Pause*] OK. Goodbye.

[*Puts phone down*]

Gillian: [*To DA*] You can't give out any information on the phone. Ex-wife! You'll be surprised at what people do to get information about people. They lie and all sorts.

[*DA comment: I was struck by the contrast of this encounter with the open exchanges I observed on the surgical ward*]   (Field notes)

The division of labour on the ward also undermined information giving. The surgical ward was staffed by an all-qualified workforce, the majority of whom had nursing degrees, whereas the medical staff comprised a mixture of auxiliaries, students and staff nurses and enrolled nurses. Only the ward manager was a graduate. The ward frequently employed agency and bank staff who did not necessarily share the ward commitment to participatory practice. Drawing on Strauss *et al.* (1964) Davis (1980) has underlined the importance of having 'ideology bearers' in hospital settings in order to ensure implementation of caring philosophies. Moreover, it was not unusual for only one qualified member of staff to be on a shift. As a consequence, it was necessary to work with a division of labour in which the auxiliaries and students provided the hands-on care, and the qualified nurse concentrated on ward co-ordination, liaison and paperwork. There was not the same sense of ownership of patients in this setting and care was fragmented. It was the auxiliaries who had closest contact with patients and their families and, although this accorded them considerable power relative to staff nurses (see also

Chapter 2, this volume), they expressed continued frustration at their inability to respond to questions and queries as this extract from an interview indicates.

DA: One of the things that interests me is how, if you are doing most of the hands-on stuff and having most of the patient contact, what happens if people start asking you – and the nurses are dealing with the doctors and all the organising discharge and stuff – what happens if people presumably want to know stuff? Do you get asked lots of questions?

Auxiliary: Oh yes lots but at the end of the day all I can say is that 'I'm awful sorry I can't tell you, you are going to have to speak to the qualified staff. Basically we know what the answers are but we are not allowed to tell them. Because we read the notes as well so we know roughly what has been said but we are not allowed to do it.

DA: No.

Auxiliary: We probably know better – I'm not being funny but sometimes we probably know more than the actual qualified who was on that day. Like Gillian, Gillian's been off for four or five days – she don't know any of the patients down that side. But me and Pat know them all. So if someone had asked us how someone was we know what he was like yesterday, we know what he was like the day before. I think we could probably tell the relative 'Well he was a bit down today' but like all Gillian could tell her was what's going on now. Sometimes I don't think its worth telling, or telling a patient's relatives what is wrong sometimes you might as well say 'Yeah he's fine' which is wrong but there's nothing you can do about that. It's just the disadvantages of being an NA I suppose that you're not allowed to tell patients and relatives anything. You're not even allowed to tell patients anyway.

DA: So you direct them back to...

Auxiliary: You direct them back to the qualified staff, which is sometimes, is very annoying because qualified staff haven't got a clue who they are. I mean sometimes they have not got any idea who they are.

(Interview – Auxiliary)

Because of the need to cover the ward, the auxiliaries who had been caring for the patients did not routinely attend handover. Therefore, they were unable to contribute to the inter-shift transfer of information.

I'm not allowed to go in on handover. It is the qualified nurse who goes in on handover.

DA: That's interesting. It's something I've noticed and thought about.

Auxiliary: So on the sides Gillian will go in and do handover on Jack right she will say 'Jack Williams, seventy-eight, blah blah, left-sided weakness, blah blah blah – fine been fine all morning'. That's crap. The man has been fine admittedly but he was a little bit incontinent this morning, which upset him greatly. He had three bottles this morning and he will not accept anyone to help him onto the commode other than his wife. That's not going to be passed on at hand-over. He gets upset if he dirties. He gets very embarrassed if he's got marks on his pyjamas and the doctor comes – very embarrassed. That's not going to be on the handover. It's only what I know.

(Interview – Auxiliary)

I frequently overheard qualified staff admit to 'not knowing the patient' and witnessed them having to consult the medical notes in order to deal with an inquiry from family members, which did little to instil public confidence in them.

The phone rings and staff nurse answers it.

Staff nurse: Medical ward can I help you? [*Pause*]. He's my patient. Let me just consult my list. He's been a lot better since he came into hospital. No more pain. [*Pause*]. No not really. [*Pause*]. OK I'll go and let him know now. OK Bye. [*Goes off down the ward*].   (Fieldnotes)

Workload

The medical ward was also much busier than the surgical ward. Turnover was rapid and the beds were frequently rearranged in order to accommodate new admissions, which thwarted the nurses' aims. Unlike the surgical ward, the nurses were not proactive in information giving. For the most part there was insufficient time. Information leaflets were available on the ward but these were used sporadically, often simply added to the clutch of paperwork patients were discharged home with. Moreover, because the ward was so busy, patients and their families found it difficult to find the right moment to approach staff with their questions and so experienced considerable uncertainty, which caused anxiety. Patients complained that the nurses were too busy to talk to them and families expressed concerns that their loved ones would be unable to make their needs known to the nurses if they were not there to undertake 'advocacy work' (Allen 2000c; see also Chapter 8, this volume) on their behalf.

During the course of the fieldwork one relative lodged a formal complaint because her husband had not had his hygiene needs met by the time she arrived on the ward at 10:00 a.m. This complaint in part stemmed from her anxieties about the standards of care possible given the staffing levels, but also from the failure of nursing staff to communicate the reasons for the delay to the patient. As the nurse later explained to me:

> *Staff nurse*: There were only two of us on Saturday morning. I had to send Sally off sick – she looked absolutely awful and I thought something awful was going to happen to her so I sent her off at about 9 o'clock. So there was just Mary (auxiliary) and I. I thought we were doing well and then we had a complaint because a patient was not washed by 10 o'clock.
>
> *DA*: From a patient or relatives?
>
> *Auxiliary*: Relatives. I tried to explain the reasons why but I couldn't because everything I could say just sounded as if I was making excuses. I explained that there were only two of us and that I was the only qualified on and that there were things that I had to do but she didn't want to know she kept saying 'Oh I've heard it all before'. We'd done everybody else and about ten past eleven we went to this patient – I knew he was the sort of patient who would be 'Ten millimetres to the left and a centimetre to the right' – which is fine – but I wanted to leave myself the time to do him. So we went up to him to start his wash and the wife said 'I washed him'! So I said 'Oh well thank you very much'. And then she said that she felt that he'd been totally neglected. I said that that was not the case and that he'd had his breakfast and we'd made sure that he'd been given a drink. (Fieldnotes)

Because of the skill mix and busyness of the ward, routines were much in evidence. When workloads are onerous, routinisation is one way in which staff can ensure that everyone receives a minimal level of care (see also Chapter 2, this volume). A corollary of this, however, is that it leaves little room for flexibility and can result in individual needs being ignored or denied.

> A relative comes out to the ward corridor from the nine-bedded area.
>
> *Relative*: He needs the toilet.
>
> *DA*: OK we'll be there. [*To staff nurse*] Mr [name] wants the toilet.
>
> *Staff nurse*: He's got a pad.
>
> *Relative*: [*Has come right out to the nurses' station*]: He wants to go to the toilet.
>
> *Staff nurse*: He's just been.
>
> *Relative*: [*Looks at clock*] Well I've been here an hour and he's not been.

Staff nurse: He went when we washed him.

Relative: He's insistent that he wants to go.

Staff nurse: He's got a pad in.

Relative: He says he wants to go.

Staff nurse: OK – we'll be there – give me a minute – it will need three of us [*Returns to filling in the form she was writing. She continues writing for sometime – too long in my view*]

DA: Do you want a hand?

Staff nurse: We need three.   (Fieldnotes)

SEN: How are you?
[*The patient is sitting on the side of the bed. He is wearing a pyjama jacket but no trousers*]

Patient: I want to get back to bed.

SEN: You'll be having breakfast in a minute so you can stay there if you put that blanket over you.
[*SEN covers the patient's knees over*]
[*Patient groans*]

SEN: You've got a cup of tea there. Can you manage it? [*Hands cup to patient who takes it but says nothing*].   (Fieldnotes)

Morale

The pressures of the work environment clearly had a deleterious effect on staff morale. The ward manager complained that she spent all her time avoiding complaints and, when asked to characterise how the ward team saw themselves, most described themselves as 'the put upon ward'. This contrasts with the surgical ward where staff deployed adjectives such as 'dynamic', 'nursing development unit', and 'forward looking'. Medical ward morale had indirect effects on the quality of care. Because of the relentless slog, staff chose to use quieter periods to regenerate their batteries and socialise, rather than using the time to give patients 'the little extras' which make the difference between acceptable and good quality care (Attree 2001).

I think that the pressure is so constant on here at the moment that you are pushed really to do the things you know that have to be done. So as you say when you do get an extra couple of minutes you sort of think 'Oh well we've done quite well this morning yeah we'll have a cup of tea and then it's going to be time to do the Bs and then it's lunch sort of thing'. (Interview – Staff nurse)

During the fieldwork a number of the families I talked to expressed the view that they were considering lodging a complaint about the staffing levels on the ward. Certain staff nurses, felt that this would be one way of drawing hospital managers' attention to their difficulties, and supported them. The medical ward nurses displayed emotional detachment more often than on the surgical ward, where this was rarely evident. Allan (2001) has noted that nurses disengage from patients when they have other pressing work concerns. All too frequently on the medical ward staff had insufficient resources to accomplish the highly visible work of meeting patients' physical and technical needs, let alone find time to emotionally connect with patients and their families. One of the most uncomfortable aspects of my fieldwork role was having to witness users' anxiety, distress and frustration whilst at the same time recognising that the staff nurses were hugely overworked and simply did not have time to spend with them. In many instances I played an important mediating role, explaining the situation to patients and their families on the one hand and drawing their distress to the attention of the nursing staff on the other.

I seated myself back in the nine-bedded area. The two male visitors are coming back from the toilets with the new patient. They are supporting him – walking either side of him. He is now wearing a hospital gown. When they reach his bed the two female relatives stand up and move back so they can get through.

Male relative: Come on Bob. Which side did you want to get in? [*The patient is turning to the right even though it is the left-hand side of the bed where the covers are folded back*]. Is this side better for you?

Female relative: He prefers to get in this side. [*Adjusts the bed covers. The two men walk the patient to the right-hand side of the bed. They take his trousers down*].

Male relative: OK Bob we'll just get these off for you. Hold on a minute. [*The patient sits on the side of the bed. One of the female relatives takes his socks off*].

Female relative: I'll take your socks off.

[*The patient mutters something inaudible*].

Female relative: You don't want them on: it's too hot in here.

[*The two men help Bob into bed. They sit him up the bed and replace his oxygen mask.*]

Male relative: [*Putting oxygen mask on the patient*]. That's it. You keep that on.

[*Meanwhile the women are sorting out his clothes*]

Female relative: What should I do with his trousers? Take them home?

Male relative: You can just put them in his locker there.

[*The relatives have a pair of hospital pyjama bottoms they have not used. One of the female relatives is wandering around unsure what to do with them. The male relative takes them from her and puts them on the trolley in the corridor. The family wants to leave but they haven't spoken to the staff nurse yet and they are concerned that Bob still does not have a call bell that they requested earlier. From my vantagepoint on the ward I can see that they are not very happy. They are looking anxiously around the ward and muttering amongst themselves. Staff nurse is admitting another patient at the end of the ward and the student and auxiliary are laughing and joking over a cup of tea at the nurses' station. I feel conspicuous – I know the family want attention – and in their eyes I must appear to be doing nothing. I cannot sit back and watch this any longer. I feel compelled to intervene before this situation gets worse. I went out to see the auxiliary and the student nurse. I asked if they had a call bell organised for the new patient. The auxiliary nodded to the one lying on the desk.*]

DA: Can I take this?

Auxiliary: Yes.

DA: Where do I put it.

Auxiliary: Just plug it in.

DA: Where?

Auxiliary: In the wall next to the emergency buzzer.

DA: Did you see the relatives lifting him up the bed earlier.

Auxiliary: Well they're very silly. They should ask for help.

DA: I think they did but no one came.

[*I took the call bell into the nine-bedded area*]

DA: Were you waiting for this? Sorry – I was eavesdropping. [*I plugged in the call bell and placed it on the bed beside the patient*] [*To the patient*] If you want the nurse Bob you can press this.

Female relative: He's confused and deaf he won't hear you. [*Raises voice*] Here's your bell Bob. Press that if you want the nurse. [*To me*] He probably won't use it but the man there [*Nodding to the patient in the next bed*] said he would keep an eye on him.

DA: The other patients are very good. They all look after each other.

Female relative: Do they?

DA: Oh yes. Were you wanting to go?

Female relative: We were waiting to see the nurse.

DA: Yes I'm sorry she's very busy tonight. She's the only qualified nurse on duty. I'll have a word.

[*I wandered down the ward and whispered to the staff nurse that I thought they were getting a bit frustrated. Staff nurse said she would be with them very shortly*].

DA: [*To relative*] She's nearly finished with the gentleman at the end and then she'll be with you.   (Fieldnotes)

Participatory caring contexts and ward 'shape'

Thus far I have concentrated on how resource issues impacted upon the ability of the two ward staffs to create a participatory caring environment. As we have seen, these effects were both direct and indirect. These findings resonate with those of Savage (1995) who has observed how similar philosophies of care can be expressed differently because of differences in resources and case mix. There was, however, a further factor, quite unrelated to resources, which also contributed to the differences I have outlined: ward 'shape' (Strauss *et al.* 1985).

For the most part the surgical ward dealt with elective cases admitted with a limited number of conditions. Because they were undergoing surgery, the general health of the patient-population was relatively high and because the surgery was elective, their care was predictable. The patient population on the medical ward was much more variable. Many of the patients admitted to the ward had multiple medical problems and complex health and social care needs. Their overall levels of health were poorer. Even if the resources had been the same on both wards, the medical nurses faced greater challenges than their surgical counterparts in realising their aspirations for participatory practice. It was relatively easy for surgical nurses to provide information and answer fully patients' questions because their trajectories of care could be known with some certainty. This was not the case on the medical ward.

Strauss *et al.* (1985) use the metaphor of 'shape' to refer to the typical conditions treated on a ward. These are the routine cases for whom the tasks are known and the work organisation well understood. When patients are admitted to a ward with an illness or condition that does not fit the ward shape then problems arise. This was true of the surgical ward. Over the fieldwork period I encountered two patients who did not fit the typical cases normally admitted to the ward. In both instances, these patients were less happy with the quality of the information they had received than the majority view I have described here. Yet, it was rarely possible to predict the care of people admitted to the medical ward. Moreover, because there was acute pressure on medical beds across the Directorate the medical ward frequently accommodated other consultant's patients. 'Outliers' added an additional layer of complexity with which staff had to contend. They were often unfamiliar with the consultant concerned, and the nurses complained that the medical team saw them less frequently, making communication and information-giving even more challenging. It seems likely therefore, that because the 'shape' of the surgical ward was relatively fixed, creating a participatory caring context was always likely to be easier compared to the medical ward.

Hospital skill mixes are predicated on models of care which render much of nursing work invisible. Because medical patients often require high levels of physical tending but relatively low levels of technology, staffing levels are calculated in order to ensure sufficient pairs of hands. Surgical staffs tend to be skill rich because of the assumed technical demands of caring for post-operative patients. This completely overlooks the consequences of dilution for the organisation of the work, information giving and communication and staff morale.

Three years after the completion of the fieldwork a review of nursing establishment figures in the Medical Directorate was undertaken in response to concerns raised both internally and externally. Standard workload measurement tools for assessing skill mix were rejected as unreliable. Instead, data was generated through a number of sources: (i) a snapshot assessment of what work was not done at the end of a sample of shifts; (ii) interviews with ward managers; (iii) identification of insufficient staffing; (iv) workload assessment of ward managers; (v) workload assessment of qualified and unqualified nurses; (vi) organisation of the ward environment and (vii) quality indicators. The report recommended a 3-year plan to improve the establishment numbers on the wards in the Medical Directorate. Central to this was recognition of the need to improve the staffing levels and increase the ratio of qualified to unqualified staff.

Conclusion

In this chapter I have examined how staff on two wards accomplished the context of care. I have argued that orthodox analyses of the lay–professional interface in the nursing context have over-emphasised the importance of individual relationships, neglecting exploration of how features of the caring environment contribute to or detract from participatory practice.

Participatory models of practice in nursing were ushered in on a wave of consumerism, which has flowed through health policies over the past twenty years. There is no evidence of any change of direction in recent government policy; in fact, if anything consumerism is becoming even more marked. Much has been made of the need for culture changes and health service staffs are frequently berated for their conservatism. Whilst we may not embrace fully the new models of patient-hood present in the policy and professional literature, it is also clear that the creation of a participatory caring environment requires sufficient resources to make it happen. Moreover, these findings indicate that there is a need for a review of skill-mix formulae in order to take into account the work involved in creating a participatory caring context, which has hitherto remained invisible. Retention and recruitment of nursing staff is currently a key government concern. If adequate resources do not match raised public expectations, there is a real danger that more nurses will become increasingly frustrated and vote with their feet.

> There's nothing the nurses can do to make the patients feel more able to ask them things when the patients repeatedly tell me how busy the nurses are. [...] The patients [...] do not want to impose on the nurses in asking them to do things relating to their basic care let alone request more information. (Fieldnotes)

8 Negotiating the role of *expert carers* on an adult hospital ward

Davina Allen

Introduction

Owing to a combination of economic, demographic and ideological factors, the last 20 years has witnessed the 'rediscovery' of family care (Nolan *et al.* 1996). Apart from notable exceptions, such as Sweden (Hokenstad and Johansson 1990; cited by Zarit *et al.* 1993), contemporary systems of welfare are increasingly underpinned by the assumption that families or significant others should care for their dependent relatives. There has been a concomitant explosion of research into caring over the past decade. We now have a better understanding of the incidence, patterns and experience of family caregivers (Twigg and Atkin 1994), the sorts of help carers say they need and the temporal elements of the care-giving career (Taraborrelli 1994; Nolan *et al.* 1996). Much less is known, however, about how carers fit into the service system. The aim of this chapter is to begin to address this gap in the literature by exploring the ways in which staff on an adult medical ward negotiated the caring division of labour with *established* family carers. I refer to this group as *expert carers* and argue for their analytic distinction from other family members or significant others who may have been implicated in the ward caring division of labour in some way. The argument presented here is that in terms of our understanding of the negotiation of the caring division of labour in the hospital context expert carers constitute a special case because of the challenge they pose to fundamental features of the social organisation of work on the wards.

The changing boundary between formal and informal care: policy background

In the UK, changes in the division of labour between formal and informal carers have to be understood in terms of the politics of community care. The idea of community care first emerged in the context of the 1959 Mental Health Act and rapidly became common currency in relation to a whole range of client groups. Initially, the emphasis was on care 'in' the community, but during the 1970s this began to shift and care 'by' the community became a much more prominent feature of public policy (Finch 1990). These policy trends reflected a number of different pressures: an ageing population, public expenditure contraction and a coming together of left-wing critiques of the repressive nature of institutional care and right-wing policies which emphasised self-help and the importance of the family. By the end of the decade informal family care had become a central plank of service provision.

These broader trends have found expression within nursing. Contemporary nursing ideologies emphasise the importance of involving family and friends in the care of their significant others (e.g. Wilson 1993; Buckwalter *et al.* 1993; Orem 1995). Family care is implicitly accepted as a 'good thing', empowering the client and protecting against feelings of helplessness (e.g. Brooking 1989), improving compliance and supporting early hospital discharge (e.g. Meyer 1993).

Lay experts and the caring division of labour

Given the sustained social scientific interest in family carers in recent years, it is surprising that so little sociological attention has been given to their involvement in the caring division of labour on hospital wards. This may, in part, reflect the existence of disciplinary divisions within the literature. Apart from a few notable exceptions (Nolan *et al.* 1996), there has been relatively little cross-fertilisation between nursing and the social sciences in this substantive area. As I have indicated, for the most part, it is the positive aspects of informal care-giving that have been emphasised in the nursing context. Much of the writing within sociology and social policy, however, has been undertaken from within a feminist perspective and has tended to concentrate on care-giving within the domestic division of labour. This work has been mainly critical of how the assumptions that underpin family care are exploitative of women (e.g. Finch 1990; Ungerson 1990).

The one notable exception to this overall dearth in the sociological literature is the study by Rosenthal *et al.* (1980) of the relationship between nurses, patients and their families on four acute care wards in a Canadian teaching hospital. Employing a negotiated order perspective, the book as a whole emphasises the problem of conflict and describes itself as a study of dilemmas in care and control. Rosenthal *et al.* (1980) argue that lay people and health professionals come from two different worlds and bring to the hospital setting different definitions of the situation and different goals. Nurses, like other workers, seek to control the conditions of their work, whereas patients and their families seek to control the conditions of their hospital experience. Negotiation of control takes place in a situation of unequal power.

The authors suggest that in order to control family members, hospital nurses cast them into one of three roles. Drawing on Glaser and Strauss (1965), Rosenthal *et al.* (1980) argue that the most common role for family members is the 'visitor' role. This is the preferred role they argue, because it is most familiar and least threatening to nurses' control over the work. The role of 'worker' is imputed in the case of relatives who are becoming increasingly involved in aspects of the patient's care. In this instance, the relative has been brought into the authority system and has been placed in a subordinate position. Nurses may also cast family members into the 'patient' role. According to Rosenthal *et al.* (1980), this may happen if the worker role starts to break down and the nurse wishes to reassert her authority.

Rosenthal *et al.* (1980) provide a useful starting point. Yet, despite the authors' claims about the study's focus, families actually receive scant attention in the book (one chapter out of six). Moreover, their analysis is derived from data generated in meetings, hence there is little evidence of the processes through which hospital staff and family members negotiate their roles. Crucially, for the purposes of this paper, families are treated as a homogeneous group. My data suggest that this is not the case. Rather, it indicates the existence of a distinct group of family carers referred to in this paper as expert carers who, for analytic purposes, need to be distinguished from other informal caregivers who may be involved in the provision of care in the hospital context. The key difference is that expert carers have an *established* care-giving relationship with a relative or loved one.

The literature suggests that for established family-caregivers, care is both an activity and an identity (Lewis and Meredith 1988; Taraborrelli 1994). Carers develop a strong sense of responsibility for the cared-for and over the course of their care-giving careers develop considerable expertise (Taraborrelli 1994; Twigg and Atkin 1994; Nolan *et al.* 1996). The expert carer, like the 'expert patient' (MacIntyre and Oldman 1977), develops a special knowledge of the cared-for person's needs, derived from their particular circumstances and from their experience of the way in which the person they are caring for responds to their illness experience. In this paper I argue that this constellation of features marks expert carers out from other family members who may be involved in caring processes on hospital wards and makes their integration into the division of labour potentially problematic.

The study

The data employed in this study are drawn from wider research into the ways in which nurses, patients and their friends and family negotiated care. The study was undertaken on a medical ward and a surgical ward in a large UK university teaching hospital. As there were no examples of expert carers on the surgical ward, only the material generated on the medical ward is examined here. These data comprise: fieldnotes arising from two months as a participant observer of the social worlds of nurses, health care assistants, patients and their carers; tape-recorded interviews with a sample of ward staff (four auxiliaries and nine qualified nurses) and extended, non-tape-recorded interviews with eleven patients and six carers, which, as far as it was possible, were recorded contemporaneously. Interviews lasted from 30 minutes to one hour (a full account of the study's method can be found in Chapter 7).

Expert carers and the caring division of labour on the ward

Consistent with contemporary nursing ideology, the inclusion of family members in the caring division of labour was generally encouraged in the study site. 'Family involvement' was a stated aim of the ward philosophy although the form this should take was not specified. Nevertheless, in their accounts of their work, the nurses and auxiliaries used the notion of 'family involvement' to refer to strategies aimed at reducing the traditional asymmetries between healthcare providers and the general public – such as improved communications – and also the inclusion of family and friends in the physical tasks of caring. The ward had an open visiting policy:[13] family and friends were permitted to visit the unit at any time. Staff also underlined the importance of communication and information-giving, although at times the exigencies of the work meant this fell short of their ideals (see also Chapter 7, this volume). This provided the context against which the involvement of family and significant others was negotiated.

As I have suggested, informal carers are not a homogeneous group. Owing to their prior care-giving experience established family carers constitute a distinct category of carer. In order to make this distinction more explicit, it is necessary to provide an overview of the involvement of family members on the ward in general before moving on to explicate the case of expert carers in particular. Although they provide relatively little data to substantiate their descriptive categories Rosenthal *et al.* (1980) do provide a useful starting point for exploring the immersion of family members in the caring division of labour on the ward. Setting aside the patient role for current purposes, the visitor and worker roles outlined by Rosenthal *et al.* (1980) capture the range of family involvement in caring work found on the ward in this study.

'Visitors'

Families' immersion in the ward division of labour was highly variable. The 'visitor' represents the least involved extreme, although this was not an entirely passive role as Rosenthal *et al.* (1980) suggest. In the wards studied 'visitors' did contribute to the caring division of labour but this work was largely taken-for-granted by nursing staff, possibly because these activities were considered to be a legitimate element of normal affective relations between kin and friends. Caring tasks undertaken by 'visitors' included: tidying the bedside area, pouring drinks, basic 'comfort work' (Strauss *et al.* 1985) such as rearranging pillows and bed-covers, making the patient's needs known to ward staff, accompanying the patient off the ward, keeping a watchful eye on the patient's safety, and providing recreational activities.

'Workers'

The 'worker' role is located at the opposite end of the continuum of family involvement in care. Family members who negotiated a 'worker role', immersed themselves in the ward division of labour in ways which went beyond the taken-for-granted activities which constitute the reciprocity of normal affective relationships. For example, they undertook certain technical procedures, intimate tending and body products work. Their involvement in caring work appeared to be both patient and nurse-oriented. In addition to undertaking care-giving for the benefits of their loved ones, workers were also concerned to be of help to the ward staff. Those adopting the worker role were the subject of friendly banter.

> *Wife*: Julie said to me 'We'll just get you some trousers and a top and you can join the team.'   (Fieldnotes)

I have used the visitor and worker roles to describe the range of family involvement in caring *activities* on the ward. Within this there was considerable variation in the extent to which family members and significant others were engaged with the details of the patient's condition, that is, the extent to which nurses used them as a legitimate source of information about the client or granted them information about the case.

Expert carers

Like the 'workers', expert carers tended to spend long periods of time on the ward and undertook care-giving work that went beyond the taken-for-granted activities associated with normal affective relations. They were also closely involved with the details of the patient's case. But whereas, relatives and friends who adopted a 'worker' role remained subordinate members of the workforce, expert carers were more oriented to the needs of the patient, rather than the nurses, and as a consequence their actions could lead them to disrupt fundamental features of the social organisation of ward work. Expert carers presented important challenges to the ward nurses' ability to control the work, their claims to expertise and their licence (Hughes 1984) to define standards of nursing care. Thus, whilst other family members could be integrated into the ward caring division of labour with relative ease, the integration of expert carers was infinitely more problematic.

The analysis that follows is based on the four cases of expert carers and their loved ones encountered over the period of the study. In two of the cases the expert carers were wives caring for dependent spouses, one case was a son caring for his frail elderly mother, and the other was a family of expert carers who shared the caring burden between them, although it was the wife who actually lived with her dependent husband and who carried responsibility for his care. All the patients had been admitted to hospital in response to a crisis situation, and, with one exception, the admission had raised questions about the family's ability to care for their relative in their home environment. Thus for at least three of the families in the study, negotiation of the caring division of labour was taking place at the same time as they were also wrestling with the need to 'let go'. Although, these emotions were rarely made explicit, they formed a crucial part of the wider context against which care was negotiated (Strauss 1978; Sugrue 1982). Almost all of the incidents of conflict and difficulty I observed at the boundary between formal–informal carers were in relation to these particular cases.

Negotiating responsibility and control

My conversations with expert carers indicated that they had a very strong sense of responsibility for their relatives. Although they may have delegated some of the care-giving work to ward staff, their sense of ownership remained. Compared to the home situation, however, the expert carer on the ward has far less control over the caring process (Ungerson 1990) and this caused immense frustration and was a significant point of tension with ward staff.

> *Mrs Durham*: There's supposed to be such a thing as visitor power and when people are here they are supposed to be able to be involved in care. *So how do I get a doctor to see my husband?* I'm really worried about him. He's not eaten for twenty-four hours and I think someone should come and see him.
>
> *DA*: Have you spoken to the nurses about this?
>
> *Mrs Durham*: Repeatedly but I don't seem to be able to get anyone to come.
>
> *DA*: I know they were waiting for someone to come to put the tube down.
>
> *Mrs Durham*: My husband thinks that they are starving him and that they don't care about him because he is old. He's very depressed and I have to be here the whole time – and it's just as well I can be – which is tiring and very stressful.
> [...]
> *[A staff nurse joins us]*
>
> *Mrs Durham*: Where is the doctor? Why haven't they come and seen him?
>
> *Staff nurse*: It was the on-call doctor. She was on late last night and she's had to do the post-take ward round this morning.
>
> *Mrs Durham: But they said that they would be here!*
>
> *Staff nurse*: We put a lot of fine bore tubes down because they come out a lot – if the patient sneezes or rolls over – so we have to put a lot down. It may not have been given a very high priority.
>
> *Mrs Durham*: But they've stopped him eating. That can't be good.
>
> *Staff nurse*: That's because they were concerned that it would go into his lungs.
>
> *Mrs Durham*: I know but not feeding him can't be doing him any good.

Staff nurse: It's better than feeding him.

Mrs Durham: Well that's a matter of opinion. If they don't put a tube down I shall start feeding him again myself.

Staff nurse: But you risk him having a chest infection – which could be fatal.

Mrs Durham: But not feeding him can't be doing him any good.

Staff nurse: Going without food for a few hours won't do any harm but if he eats and it goes into his lungs it could be fatal. I'm sorry if it all appears a bit casual to you but.

Mrs Durham: Yes it does *[walks off down the corridor]*.

Staff nurse [To DA]: You see what I mean?

DA: It's very difficult.   (Fieldnotes – original emphasis)

As well as illustrating the frustration and giving some indication of the fear engendered by expert carers' loss of control over the caring process, this extract also provides a vivid example of *advocacy work*. I have used this concept to refer to the work undertaken by family and friends in making the needs of their relatives known to nurses. Clearly, not all the examples were this dramatic, nevertheless caregivers' attempts to exert some control over the care-giving process by undertaking advocacy work were an on-going source of strain.

Auxiliary: Sometimes they've [family carers] got no patience. If they ask for something they want it yesterday. [...] If I'm in the nine-bedded ward I've got another eight patients to think about. So you've got to just grit your teeth and smile. [Laughs] (Interview – Auxiliary)

She's here all the time and I don't think its doing her any good. She's got nothing to do so she's complaining about this, that and the other. (Fieldnotes – Staff nurse)

Priorities and perspectives

As I described in Chapter 7 the medical ward was very busy. Although the nurses were supportive of the principle of involving family and friends in the caring division of labour, implementing this in practice placed additional demands on their limited time and undermined their work control. Arguably part of the problem, as Hughes (1984) points out, is that in nursing, as in many areas of work, the work of one person is frequently made up of the emergencies of another.

Hughes characterises the relationship between routines and emergency as in a state of chronic tension. The person with the crisis feels that the other is trying to belittle their trouble, however the worker's claim to competence arises from having dealt with many similar cases. As we have seen, related to this is the struggle to maintain some decisions over what work to do, and over the disposition of one's time and one's routine of life. A further difficulty relates to differences in the priorities and perspectives of ward staff and family members. Expert carers, understandably, were primarily concerned with the needs of their loved one, whereas nurses had to focus on the needs of the entire ward.

> It was horrendous on here on Monday. One of the patients went for a CT [scan] and had an arrest [cardiac arrest] when he was down there. His family were on the ward waiting for him. His grandchildren and everything. They got him back [successfully resuscitated him] and he came back to the ward. It was awful – the grandson threw himself on him and wouldn't let him go. The physio came to give him some suction and he arrested again. I went to get his family in again. He took another two breaths and died. They were all terribly upset. They wanted to spend some time with him so I took the grandchildren out of the way for them. Mrs Durham saw me with them and got upset. She said 'You'd rather look after those children than care for my husband. You don't care about him'. (Fieldnotes – Staff nurse)

Misunderstandings of this kind are extremely difficult for the nurses to deal with. If they do not justify their actions the accusation stands unchallenged and threatens the breakdown of relationship with the expert carer. If they do explain the situation to the family carer-giver then they risk compounding the emotional distress of the family member by pointing out the inappropriateness of their complaint.

Negotiating expertise

As I have noted, over the course of their care-giving career carers develop considerable caring knowledge. Drawing on Harvath *et al.* (1994), Nolan *et al.* (1996) contrast the local knowledge of family carers with the global and generic knowledge of formal carers. Harvath *et al.* (1994) suggest that it is the skilful blending of the local knowledge of family caregivers with the generic knowledge of formal carers which results in the most profitable interaction between carers and service providers. Arguably, however, this is easier said then done: negotiation of expertise in the hospital context is underpinned by a number of important tensions.

Participatory practice and claims to profession

One such tension relates to the difficulties ward nurses face in reconciling two contradictory elements within contemporary nursing ideology: the rhetoric of participatory practice which includes informal carers and the client, and the claim to professional status and expertise. As Hughes points out: 'Professionals *profess*. They profess to know better than others the nature of certain matters, and to know better than their clients what ails them. This is the basis of their license' (Hughes 1984: 375). The fragility of nurses' jurisdictional claims has been well-documented (e.g. Dingwall *et al.* 1988; Davies 1994; Rafferty 1996). Historically, one of the main obstacles to nurses achieving professional status is that most nursing tasks are undertaken by unqualified care-givers: paid auxiliaries and care-assistants or unpaid carers. A further difficulty relates to the fact that although at one level certainly nurses' knowledge is global and generic compared to the local knowledge of expert carers, contemporary nursing ideology also lays special claim to an individualised and holistic approach to care based on the nurse–patient relationship (Salvage 1992). 'Knowing the patient' is an important element of nurses' occupational identity and central to their sense of professional competence (Allen 1998; also see Chapter 2, this volume). In negotiating the caring division of labour on the wards nurses are caught between the dual pressures of the need to recognise the expertise of established carers and their aspirations to accomplish profession (Dingwall 1977).

Although nurses recognised that family caregivers were a valuable resource, they found it difficult to draw on this knowledge in a way that did not undermine their sense of professional competence.

Staff nurse: I think we could learn from the carers who've looked after them for years at home – the best ways to manage them, the best ways to move them or we could take a lot more input from them.

DA: Why don't you?

Staff nurse: I don't really know. I don't know why it's not done. I suppose it's everybody's way of looking at it – you don't want to admit you don't know. By asking for help you are almost admitting a failure – that there's a little bit of you – you don't want to be seen by the relatives as not being able to cope with their friend or relative or whoever it is. (Fieldnotes)

It was rare for nurses to pro-actively solicit the advice and opinion of expert carers. As a consequence it was extremely difficult for family and relatives to make a positive contribution without this being interpreted as a criticism.

Lawler (1991) suggests that one way in which nurses have managed their vulnerability to criticism or interference from relatives and visitors is by asking them to leave when they provide body care for patients. However, in keeping with contemporary nursing ideology, most of the nurses allowed family members to be present when they attended to their loved ones. I observed only one instance in which a visitor was asked by a nurse to leave and this stood out as highly unusual. At the same time, however, having relatives and family members observing their care-giving practices clearly left nurses feeling exposed, particularly unqualified staff who, unlike professional nurses, could not lay claim to officially sanctioned expertise.

Auxiliary: [W]hen you're trying to do things for them and they're nit-picking and it's 'Oh we don't do it this way and you should be doing it that way' and 'Why hasn't the doctor been up?' And you find yourself thinking 'Oh we're doing our best'. Or turning them 'Oh he's not comfortable'. (Interview – Auxiliary)

Yeah and his wife used to stay in all the time as well. I mean obviously there's never enough room behind those curtains anyway and to have her there you know saying 'Do this' and 'Don't forget to do this' and you think 'Ahh – just leave me to it'. [*Laughs*] (Interview – Auxiliary)

Often the practices expert carers had developed at home were different from those utilised by staff on the ward and this could also cause tension.

She wants us to treat him the same as she did when he was at home. So she says 'If you ask him to put his arm there, he'll push himself up on the chair'. When I'm lifting stroke patients I like to hold them like this. [*Demonstrates a face to face handling technique with both arms round the patient*]. I like them to be in the same plane as me so I'm not having to reach round to sort out the chair. (Fieldnotes – Staff nurse)

Family caregivers, for their part, appeared to be caught between the conflicting demands of the normative expectations of the lay–professional relationship and their sense of moral responsibility for their loved ones. In their routine interactions with nursing staff, expert carers – like other family members and friends who spent time on the ward – were oriented to nurses' professional expertise and their status as the arbiter of the ward rules. For example, they talked about being careful not to 'over-step the mark' and checked with the nurses before undertaking tasks that they would have carried out without a second thought in the domestic setting. In their discussions with me, expert carers revealed that they were well aware of the risk of offending nurses' occupational identities.

> *Relative*: Well Geoff's been out again to tell them about the food but we wonder 'Do they think we're pushy, over-protective or fussy'. I don't want them to feel that we've come in and tried to take over.
>
> (Fieldnotes – Daughter-in-Law)

Carers' continuing sense of responsibility for their loved ones was strong, however, and on a number of occasions this resulted in some very direct challenges to the expertise of ward staff.

Challenging professional expertise: the case of Mrs Durham

In the extended extract I have used in my discussion of 'negotiating responsibility and control', we can see that Mrs Durham quite openly challenges the expertise of the staff nurse about the costs and benefits of not feeding her husband. This was part of an on-going disagreement between the expert carer and the hospital staff as to whether the patient should be artificially fed or not. The patient, John, had sustained a stroke and had difficulty swallowing. This had resulted in food and drink entering his lungs, causing pneumonia. At one point during the fieldwork, the medical staff believed that feeding

John normally was no longer possible and that he required an artificial feeding tube. Mrs Durham resisted this idea firmly however, despite the pressure being applied by ward staff.

> The other day there were a whole group of them there – the speech therapist, physio, a couple of nurses and some others that I didn't know – and they'd come to try and persuade me to let him have the P.E.G [artificial feeding tube]. They seemed to want me to make a decision right away and I didn't want to so I said, 'You can all go away and I will think about it'. A little later a nurse came back on the same deposition (sic). In the end I went home and I telephoned my GP, who I know and trust, and he explained it all to me and why he felt I should let the experts guide me. (Fieldnotes – Mrs Durham)

This extract vividly illustrates Mrs Durham's social isolation and highlights one way in which negotiations in the hospital setting are weighted in favour of service providers. In the end Mrs Durham did agree to the feeding tube but later, after her husband had pulled it out, she asked for a second opinion.

> I asked for a second opinion from the older speech therapist because the younger one kept on insisting he couldn't eat and I wondered if the older would be less cautious. (Fieldnotes – Mrs Durham)

Theoretically, by requesting a second opinion expert carers can question the expertise of healthcare providers. However, in practice, it is unlikely that the professional approaches the case from a position of total moral neutrality because they already have some knowledge of the history of events and are thus able to 'stage' their negotiations with carers (Levy 1982). Staging refers to the use of self-serving strategies by which individuals and groups are able to control the context in which negotiations occur. This reflects a further important way in which the negotiation context of the hospital setting augments the power of healthcare workers *vis-à-vis* the general public.

In John Durham's case a compromise was eventually reached. A decision was taken not to feed him artificially with the proviso that he should only receive thickened fluids and pureed food to minimise the risk of further respiratory complications. The speech and language therapist left written instructions as to how John should be fed. Mrs Durham also devised her own instructions, however, which she believed to be superior to those provided by the speech and language therapist.

Mrs Durham has left a note of instructions for feeding John for a meal on Monday evening. She begins by saying how much she thinks John is likely to want to eat.

Mrs Durham: I could have written more but I didn't think any one would read it.

DA: The speech therapist has left some very explicit instructions in the notes but I guess it would be useful to have them here for people to refer to.

Mrs Durham: But even the speech therapist wasn't feeding him properly. She was going too fast. She was giving him too much. Even three-quarters of a teaspoon is too much. She was putting it into the middle of his mouth but it's better to put it in the right hand side because the muscles are better on the right. And he needs to be told to swallow each time. (Fieldnotes)

I use this example to illustrate that direct challenges to professional expertise do occur and to give some indication of the undercurrents that can shape the negotiation of the formal–informal care-giving boundary. Clearly, expert carers do not have a monopoly on disputes of this kind, however, my data suggest that more than any other category of caregiver, it is expert carers who are likely to make these challenges explicit. This was the most dramatic example I observed during the course of the fieldwork but it was certainly not the only incident of this kind. It made for an emotionally charged atmosphere, which coloured all other interactions between the ward staff and the carer.

John Durham was eventually moved to another ward on the grounds that he had a faecal infection and needed to be cared for in a single room. Given that he was never actually nursed in isolation on the new ward (the nurses there said it was unnecessary) and that no attempt was made to move another patient on the medical ward with the same infection, one has to suspect that the nurses' motivations for moving John were not based on clinical grounds alone.

Staff nurse: Have you seen Mrs Durham lately?

DA: Are they still in?

Staff nurse: [*Rolls her eyes*] I don't know. The last I heard he was on Poppy Ward. I thought he'd come back when his clostridium was resolved.

DA: He was out on the ward before it was resolved.

Staff nurse: Oh well it was an excuse to get him into a cubicle. You need to share people like that. Don't you? (Fieldnotes)

It is not my purpose to demonise the ward staff in recounting this tale. They were extremely sympathetic to Mrs Durham's perspective, but at the same time, the on-going situation was demanding of their limited time and energy. Furthermore, the tensions that were engendered by the constant disagreements in this case meant that communication was extremely difficult. Having observed the situation from both sides over a number of days, I spent some time talking to John's daughter when she visited the ward one weekend. She referred to herself as having entered a 'battleground' and she talked of how she had had to cope with her mother 'in hysterics' on the telephone all week. Our conversation was informative and added a hitherto unacknowledged dimension to the dispute.

> And now his swallowing has gone – that's really awful. She [Mrs Durham] said that if he can't eat or drink wine then what quality of life has he got then? She's also a bit squeamish and doesn't fancy the tube into the stomach. (Fieldnotes – Daughter)

I suggest that in resisting the artificial feeding tube, Mrs Durham was fighting to preserve what she perceived to be the only thing of value in his life that her husband had left: eating and drinking. Furthermore, I suspect that owing to her 'squeamishness', she also feared that the feeding tube would make it difficult for her to care for him at home again. However, what was interesting – and distressing – about this case, was that although the ward staff were oriented to Mrs Durham's 'emotion standpoint' (Sugrue 1982) at no point were these emotions explicitly discussed. Rather, interaction between staff and expert carer was constituted at the surface level as a dispute over expertise. This meant that the question of whether Mrs Durham should continue feeding normally – in full recognition of the risks that this entailed – was never broached.

Negotiating standards

The literature on family caregivers suggest that carers develop a strong sense of responsibility for the cared-for and come to consider themselves to be the final judges of standards of care (Twigg and Atkin 1994; Nolan et al. 1996; Montenko 1988).

This can pose particular difficulties for the negotiation of the boundary between expert carers and ward nurses as key differences between the hospital and domestic settings make standards of care derived from the domestic context difficult to achieve.

Care in hospital and care at home

As James (1992a,b) points out, there are a number of important differences between domestic care and hospital care. Compared to the domestic setting, care in the hospital setting is accomplished via a complex hierarchically ordered division of labour. Many of the care-giving tasks performed by a single carer in the home are carried out by different categories of staff in the hospital context. Thus, whilst care in the domestic setting can be flexibly organised to meet the specific needs of the patient, within the hospital context this is less easy. Although the nurses in this study subscribed to an ideology of individualised patient care, in practice work was organised into routines so as to provide the optimum standard of care possible within the resources available. James employs the term 'carework' to refer to 'the negotiable tension between the principles and the skills in giving personal attention to individual patients and the routinisation necessary in any organisation' (1992b: 108).

A further difference between care in the domestic setting and care in the hospital context is that in the domestic setting an affective relationship between the carer and the cared-for is assumed. 'Caring' about someone provides the basis for 'caring for them'. In the hospital, the relationship between carer and cared-for is contractual (Melia 1983; cited by Kitson 1987), affective relations may develop (Qureshi 1990) but this is not the basis for the caring relationship. Compared to informal carers, formal carers have a mainly functional approach to caring work. Nurses' care-giving activities are designed to maximise patient independence (Kitson 1987; Brannon 1994); where possible the patient will be encouraged to do as much for themselves as they can. As Lawler (1991) has pointed out, nurses have a very 'task-specific' approach to what they regard as situations where patients need assistance. Compared to formal carers, the caring work of family members is shaped by their affective relationship with the cared-for and I suggest that care-giving tasks are performed as much for their value as a *symbol* of care, rather than being oriented to increasing their independence.

Comparative standards – a source of strain

These differences between care in the domestic context and care on the hospital ward could be a source of strain. Nurses complained that family caregivers made patients 'demanding'.

> [Y]ou get some patients they come in and they've been cared for at home everything's been done for them. They may expect you to carry on doing the same. So that's quite difficult. (Interview – Staff nurse)

> *Staff nurse 1*: He's quite demanding isn't he? He buzzed just to have a blanket over his knees.

> *Staff nurse 2*: I think the wife looks after him at home and does a lot for him.

> *Staff nurse 1*: He's lovely but by the end of the shift!
>
> (Fieldnotes – nursing hand-over)

It is the first few days in the patient's hospital career that the differences between family care and home care are most likely to be a source of tension between nurses and expert carers. There seem to be several possible reasons for this. First, the differences between domestic care and ward care appear to cause 'reality shock' in expert carers, creating considerable fear and anxiety and compounding what is already a difficult and emotionally charged situation. In three of the cases studied, family care-givers complained that their relative's needs were not being attended to (see also Chapter 7, this volume).

> *Daughter-in-Law*: We were worried about his needs. You can see he's very well cared for and when we first came in we were concerned that nobody was seeing to him immediately – we were used to doing everything straight away for him.   (Fieldnotes)

> *Mrs Baxter*: I thought it was dreadful that he hadn't been done [washed by 11 o' clock] so I did it myself.   (Fieldnotes)

Secondly, as James (1992a) has pointed out, although nurses subscribe to an ideology of individualised care, the constraints of care on hospital wards mean that in practice this amounts to finding out enough about patients to know when to interrupt the routines to attend to individual requirements. Although the nurses carried out an assessment of patient needs and preferences on admission to the unit, this was little more than a bureaucratic exercise. Rather, the real business of 'getting to know' the patient took time and arose out of day-to-day contact. Again this could lead to difficulties.

> She said that he hadn't had his teeth cleaned before breakfast and I explained that it was his first morning on the ward and that we couldn't know every patient's routine but that if he had asked we would have happily cleaned his teeth. (Interview – Staff nurse)

Even when nurses had established the individual preferences of patients the constraints of care in the hospital context could still mean they were unable to match the standards of care possible in the domestic setting.

> I mean if some relatives have very particular times about when a patient has their wash or medicine or whatever. Well you can't in a hospital setting – you can't always get to them at that time. (Interview – Auxiliary)

Despite these tensions about standards of care, privately a number of the carers appreciated that comparing the care on the wards with domestic care was unreasonable.

> *Son*: Now when I think about it a bit more I can understand it but at the time we were all very worried. You can't expect the same in a place like this when there are nine other patients to be looked after. (Fieldnotes)

Equally, a number of the nurses expressed the view that they felt the relatives were justified in complaining about the standards of care because the staffing levels on the ward meant they fell short of what they considered ideal. Reacting to a complaint made by an expert carer a staff nurse made the following comment:

> But the problem was that although I knew my side of the story I could to a certain extent I could sympathise with what she was saying. I think, I think if I was in her situation, if I had somebody that was a patient on the ward and the staffing levels were that low and the time being spent with my relative was so limited – I think I'd be worried and I wouldn't be happy and I would feel that maybe things might be overlooked that might be important. (Interview – Staff nurse)

Nevertheless, although both family-caregivers and nurses recognised the difficulties, once a complaint had been made, it sullied relationships between informal caregivers and ward staff.

> But it's a horrible atmosphere in there when they're in there now you feel as if they are watching you all the time. (Fieldnotes – Staff nurse)

Staff came to identify such family members as potential complainants and this resulted in defensive practices.

> He had a fall in the bathroom yesterday but his wife is a bit fanickerty (sic) so we've filled in an accident form – just in case. (Fieldnotes – Staff nurse)

Given the all-pervasive culture of risk within the NHS (Annandale 1996) it is not surprising that ward staff should respond in this way, but it is hardly conducive to the participatory relationships with family caregivers that nurses aspire to.

Discussion and conclusion

In this paper I have examined expert caregivers' integration into the caring division of labour on adult hospital wards. I have argued that in terms of our understanding of the informal–formal care-giving boundary, expert carers constitute a distinct group because of the challenges they present to key features of division of labour on the ward: ward staff's control of the work situation, their professional judgement and their license to set standards of care. Although the nurses in this study were broadly supportive of the involvement of family caregivers in the ward division of labour, they found it hard to involve expert carers in ways which did not undermine their professional identities and their ability to deal with the practical demands of their work. Expert caregivers' sense of moral responsibility for their loved ones was strong and handing over their care-giving functions to nursing staff challenged their sense of control over the caring process.

Moreover, as we have seen, negotiation of the formal–informal care-giving boundary took place against an emotionally-charged backdrop. Thus, whereas other family members and friends were integrated into the caring division of labour on the ward with relative ease, the involvement of expert carers was, at times, difficult.

The data examined here raise several issues of wider socio-logical significance. First, they highlight the need to include both the affective and the work component in any conceptual-isation of the caring division of labour. In the past, sociologists, adopting a feminist stance, have intentionally downplayed the relational aspects of informal care-giving in order to emphasise its status as work and to highlight the exploitative elements of welfare policy (e.g. Ungerson 1990). I have considerable sym-pathy with the political motivation behind such a stance. From an analytic perspective, however, to diminish the affective ele-ment of care is to overlook a key element of the negotiation context that is vital to understanding negotiation of the infor-mal–formal caring division of labour. As we have seen, a num-ber of the difficulties of integrating expert carers into the caring division of labour appeared to stem from the affective relationship between the carer and the cared-for.

Related to this, is the assertion by Rosenthal *et al.* (1980) and Glaser and Strauss (1965), that nurses impute the patient role to family members when their involvement in the caring division of labour becomes disruptive. There are certainly instances in my data that appear to support such a claim. However, I would caution against interpreting nurses' actions in a singularly punitive light. Even though the nurses in this study found relations with expert carers fraught at times, they nevertheless had a great deal of sensitivity to their 'emotion standpoint' and their imputation of the patient role reflected these genuine concerns as much as they did the desire to reassert control over the work process. There is clearly a need for sociological research to give further attention to the ways in which emotions shape negotiations in the healthcare con-text and indeed, how emotions may themselves be subject to negotiation.

These findings also raise some interesting questions about the nature of expert knowledge particularly in relation to recent trends in healthcare which, on the one hand emphasise the importance of partnerships with the lay public and yet, on the other, progressively dilute the formal caring workforce. As we have seen, despite advocating family involvement in the caring process and recognising informal carers' expertise, nurses found it difficult to draw on this knowledge in a way which did not undermine their professional identities. Two important issues are raised by this. First, it highlights fundamental problems with the professionalising strategy being pursued by certain nursing academics, which predicates nursing's jurisdiction claims on practitioners' unique holistic 'knowing' of the client. As we have seen, the presence of the patient's family in hospital settings creates conflicts as to who really 'knows' the patient and raises interesting questions as to whose version is to prevail. Second, these issues are magnified, in the case of support staff, who unlike qualified nurses, cannot claim access to specialist caring knowledge and who, in increasing measure are working at the front-line of service provision where negotiations with family-carers take place.

This chapter has also identified a number of ways in which care-giving is constrained by the hospital setting from the perspective of both formal and informal carers. As Rosenthal *et al.* (1980) observe, negotiations between nurses and family carers take place in a context of unequal power. In the context of this study, we have seen, for example, carers' frustration with their lack of control over the caring process and their concern not to wound nurses' professional sensibilities by being 'too interfering'. As far as family carers were concerned, the hospital was the nurses' domain.

> I asked if they minded if I came in at eleven to feed him and the staff nurse said that that would be fine. But they let you know if they want you to wait and I don't want to get in their way – *after all this is their territory and they are here to do a job. If I'm at home then that's different.* (Fieldnotes – Mrs Durham, my emphasis)

However, although at one level the balance of negotiation resources are tipped in favour of healthcare providers in the hospital context, we have also seen that formal carers are themselves constrained in important ways by the work environment. This raises the question of the effects of extra-situational constraints in shaping the negotiation of the formal–informal caring division of labour, an issue identified by Strauss (1978) in his work on the negotiated order perspective. According to Strauss the task of the researcher and that of the participants themselves is to discover just what the limits of negotiation are. My data suggest that study of the negotiation of the caring division of labour in the domestic context would yield some interesting comparative material.

Finally, some observations on generalisability and representativeness. During the course of this discussion, I have indicated that there were particular features of the ward work environment – such as staffing shortages – which may have exacerbated the challenges presented by expert carers and which resulted in some of the difficulties they posed not always being dealt with in ideal ways. One of the features of the fieldwork that I found particularly difficult was the extent to which I found myself mediating between ward staff and patients and their friends and family when relationships appeared to be in danger of breaking down. Furthermore, the cases I have presented here had all been admitted to hospital in response to a crisis of some kind. This makes for a very different backdrop to the negotiation of the informal–formal boundary compared to carers whose loved ones are admitted for respite care. Notwithstanding these considerations however, I believe that the issues that have been raised by this discussion do have a more general applicability to our understanding of the informal–formal boundary in the hospital context, although variations in case mix will mean that expert carers are more likely to be encountered on some wards than others.

Endnotes

1 The report advocates the extension of prescribing authority to a wide range of professionals, subject to the requirement that they meet certain criteria and are regularly audited. However, the authority of each new group of prescribers will only extend to a limited range of medicines, and there are proposals for a system of formal surveillance to control repeat prescribing.

2 I use the term to refer to health care assistance and auxiliaries.

3 As I have noted elsewhere (Allen 1996), the introduction of 'primary nursing' must also be understood in the context of wider professionalisation processes within nursing.

4 Porphyria is a disturbance of porphyrian metabolism characterised by an increase in the formation and excretion of porphyrins or their precursors. Sufferers may be affected by abdominal pain and gastrointestinal and neurologic disturbances.

5 Questionnaires were distributed by SETRHA. However, the telephone interviews were used by the researchers to secure the support of key personnel in some hospitals. The absence of personal contact with staff in the three non-cooperating units may well account for their reluctance to participate.

6 Questionnaires were distributed by SETRHA. However, the telephone interviews were used by the researchers to secure the support of key personnel in some hospitals. The absence of personal contact with staff in the three non-cooperating units may well account for their reluctance to participate.

7 'Qualitative questionnaire' data refers to information derived from open-ended questions and a 'comments' section on the questionnaire.

8 At the time of writing, Junior doctors' hours remain an area of concern. Acknowledging that the *New Deal* (National Health Service Executive 1991) had only been partially successful, the Government and British Medical Association recently announced a new agreement which, in line with the European Union working time directive, will cut the maximum hours junior doctors work to 48 per week over a 13-year period. Over the next three years efforts will be made to reduce all junior doctors' hours to no more than 56 hours per week (DTI 1999).

9 'Lay participation' and 'lay healthwork' are not totally satisfactory terms. They imply an inherent contrast between lay users and professional provides, and yet health professionals may themselves

be recipients of services. Conversely, health services are also provided by non-professional 'lay' staff, such as health care assistants. In the absence of a satisfactory alternative I use them as shorthand to refer to this general area of interest. I retain inverted commas in order to indicate that I employ it advisedly.

10 It should be noted that Allan (2001) also identifies the presence of 'emotional distance', which she argues was necessary for nurses to cope with the emotional costs of caring. 'Emotional awareness' and 'Emotional distance' are both aspects of the 'good enough nurse' Allan argues.

11 Whilst nurses established close relationships with patients and their families their knowledge of them was limited to that which was relevant to their care, it did not entail the kinds of surveillance as sugggested by some versions of nursing's therapeutic gaze (e.g. May 1992).

12 Outliers are those patients who are under the care of a consultant who does not have allocated beds on the ward.

13 Brooking (1989) has argued that familiarity with the ward makes the involvement of family carers more likely. Open-visiting is believed to promote greater familarity with the ward.

References

Abbott A (1988) *The System of Professions: An Essay on the Division of Expert Labor.* University of Chicago Press, Chicago.

Acheson D (1998) *Independent Inquiry into Inequalities in Health.* The Stationary Office, Norwich.

Adam B (1995) *Timewatch: The Social Analysis of Time.* Polity Press, Cambridge.

Alexander M (1990) Evaluation of a training program in breast cancer nursing. *Journal of Continuing Education in Nursing* 21(6): 260–6.

Allan H (2001) A 'good enough' nurse: supporting patients in a fertility unit. *Nursing Inquiry* 8: 51–60.

Allen D (1996) *The Shape of General Hospital Nursing: The Division of Labour at Work.* Unpublished PhD thesis, University of Nottingham.

Allen D (1997) The nursing-medical boundary: a negotiated order? *Sociology of Health and Illness* 19(4): 498–520.

Allen D (1998) Doctor–nurse relationships: accomplishing the skill-mix in health care. In Abbott P and Meerabeau L (eds) *The Sociology of the Caring Professions* (2nd edn). Taylor and Francis, London, pp. 210–33.

Allen D (2000a) 'I'll tell you what suits me best if you don't mind me saying': A sociological analysis of lay participation in health care. *Nursing Inquiry* 7(3): 182–90.

Allen D (2000b) Doing demarcation: the 'boundary-work' of nurse managers in a District General Hospital. *Journal of Contemporary Ethnography* 29(3): 326–56.

Allen D (2000c) Negotiating the role of *expert carers* on an adult hospital ward. *Sociology and Health and Illness* 22(2): 149–71.

Allen D (2001a) *The Changing Shape of Nursing Practice.* Routledge, London.

Allen D (2001b) Narrating nursing jurisdiction: 'atrocity stories' and 'boundary work'. *Symbolic Interaction* 24(1): 75–103.

Allen D and Hughes D (1993) Going for growth. *The Health Service Journal* 103(5372): 33–4.

Allen D and Lyne P (1997) Nurses' flexible working practices: some ethnographic insights into clinical effectiveness. *Clinical Effectiveness in Nursing* 1(3): 131–40.

Allen D, Griffiths L, Lyne P, Monaghan L and Murphy D (2000) *Delivering health and social care: changing roles, responsibilities and relationships.* Final report submitted to the Welsh Office of Research and Development for Health and Social Care.

Allen D, Hughes D and Pickersgill F (1993) Receptivity to expanded nursing roles: the views of junior doctors, nurses and health care assistants. Paper presented at Nurse Practitioners: The UK/USA experience conference, The Cafe Royal, London.

Annandale E (1996) Working on the front-line: risk culture and nursing in the new NHS. *Sociological Review* **44**: 416–51.

Annandale E, Clark J and Allen E (1999) *New Roles, New Responsibilities: Skill Mixes and their Implementation in Medicine and Nursing.* Final report submitted to the Department of Health Research and Development Division.

Anspach R R (1987) Prognostic conflict in life-and-death decisions: the organization as an ecology of knowledge. *Journal of Health and Social Behavior* **28**: 215–31.

Anspach R R (1993) *Deciding Who Lives: Fateful Choices: In the Intensive-Care Nursery.* University of California Press, Los Angeles.

Arber S and Gilbert N (1989) Men: the forgotten carers. *Sociology* **23**: 111–18.

Armstrong D (1983) The fabrication of nurse–patient relationships. *Social Science & Medicine* **17**(8): 457–60.

Arndt M (1994) Nurses' medication errors. *Journal of Advanced Nursing* **19**: 519–26.

Ashcroft J (1992) Rising to the challenge. Scope of practice. *Nursing Times* **88**(37): 30.

Ashworth P D, Longmate M A and Morrison P (1992) Patient participation: its meaning and significance in the context of caring. *Journal of Advanced Nursing* **17**: 1430–9.

Attree M (2001) Patients' and relatives' experiences and perspectives of 'good' and 'not so good' quality care. *Journal of Advanced Nursing* **33**(4): 456–66.

Avis M (1994) Choice cuts: an exploratory study of patients' views about participation in decision-making in a day surgery unit. *International Journal of Nursing Studies* **31**(3): 289–98.

Baker S and Lyne P (1996) Quality and patients' expectations of a surgical admission. *Seminars in Pre-operative Nursing* **5**(4): 441–7.

Ball J A and Goldstone L A (1987) *'But Who Will Make the Beds?' A Report of the Mersey Region Project on Assessment of Nurse Staffing and Support Worker Requirements for Acute General Hospitals.* Merseyside Regional Health Authority, Nuffield Institute for Health Services Studies.

Beardshaw V and Robinson R (1990) *New for Old? Prospects for Nursing in the 1990s.* Kings Fund Institute, London.

Bellaby P (1992) Broken rhythms and unmet deadlines: workers' and managers' time perspectives. In Frankenberg R (ed) *Time, Health and Medicine.* Sage, London, pp. 108–22.

Benner P E (1984) *From Novice to Expert. Excellence and Power in Clinical Nursing.* Addison Wesley, Menlo Park, CA.

Biggs S (2000) User voice, interprofessionalism and postmodernity. In Davies C, Finlay L and Bullman A (eds) *Changing Practice in Health and Social Care*. Open University Press/Sage Publications, London, pp. 366–76.

Biley F C (1992) Some determinants that effect patient participation in decision-making about nursing care. *Journal of Advanced Nursing* 17: 414–21.

Bircumshaw D (1989) A survey of the attitudes of senior nurses towards graduate nurses. *Journal of Advanced Nursing* 14: 68–72.

Bonfiglio M, Lewis J, Nesbit S and Krinsky D (1997) A contemporary perspective on pharmacy's traditional strengths. *Journal of the American Pharmaceutical Association* NS 37(6): 700–4.

Bradley C, Taylor R and Blenkinsopp A (1997) Developing prescribing in primary care. *BMJ* 314: 744–7.

Brannon R L (1994) *Intensifying Care: The Hospital Industry, Professionalization, and the Reorganization of the Nursing Labor Process*. Baywood Publishing Company, Inc., New York.

British National Formulary (BNF) (2001) *British National Formulary No.39* British Medical Association and the Royal Pharmaceutical Society of Great Britain, London.

Brooker C and Butterworth C (1991) Working with families caring for a relative with schizophrenia: the evolving role of the community psychiatric nurse. *International Journal of Nursing Studies* 28(2): 189–200.

Brooker C, Falloon I, Butterworth A, Goldberg D, Graham-Hole V and Hillier V (1994) The outcome of training community psychiatric nurses to deliver psychosocial intervention. *British Journal of Psychiatry* 165(2): 222–30.

Brooking J (1989) A survey of current practices and opinions concerning patient and family participation in hospital care. In Wilson-Barnett J and Robinson S (eds) *Directions in Nursing Research*. Scutari Press, London, pp. 97–106.

Brown C and Seddon J (1996) Nurses, doctors and the body of the patient: medical dominance revisited. *Nursing Inquiry* 3: 30–35.

Brown J S, Collins A and Duguid P (1989) Situated cognition and the culture of learning. *Educational Researcher* 18(1): 32–42.

Brownlea A (1987) Participation: myths, realities and prognosis. *Social Science & Medicine* 25(6): 605–14.

Bucher R and Stelling J (1977) *Becoming Professional*. Sage, Beverly Hills.

Buckenham J and McGrath G (1983) *The Social Reality of Nursing*. Adis Health Science Press, Baglowalah, Australia.

Buckwalter K C, Cusack D, Kruckeberg T and Shoemaker A (1993) Family involvement with communication-impaired residents in long-term care settings. In Wegner G and Alexander R (eds) *Readings in Family Nursing*. JB Lippincott, Philadelphia, pp. 208–19.

Burling T, Lentz E M and Wilson R N (1956) *The Give and Take in Hospitals: A Study of Human Organisation in Hospitals.* GP Putnams & Sons Ltd, New York.

Bury M (2001) Illness narratives: fact or fiction. *Sociology of Health and Illness* 23(3): 263–85.

Campbell-Heider N and Pollock D (1997) Barriers to physician/ nurse collegiality: an anthropological perspective. *Social Science & Medicine* 25(5): 421–5.

Caress A L (1997) Patient roles in decision making. *Nursing Times* 93(31): 45–8.

Carlisle C (1991) Post-registration degrees in nursing: a time for evaluation. *Nurse Education Today* 11: 295–302.

Caro J, Groome P and Flegel K (1993) Atrial fibrillation and anti-coagulation. *The Lancet* 341: 1381–4.

Carpenter M (1993) The subordination of nurses in health care: towards a social divisions approach. In Riska E and Wegar K (eds) *Gender, Work and Medicine.* Sage, London, pp. 95–130.

Castledine G (1992) Nursing degrees: hindrance or help? *British Journal of Nursing* 1(13): 671.

Chambliss D (1997) *Beyond Caring: Hospitals, Nurses and the Social Organization of Ethics.* University of Chicago Press, Chicago.

Chapman T (1991) The nurse's role in neuroleptic medications. *Journal of Psychological Nursing* 29(6): 6–8.

Clarke J (1999) The diminishing role of nurses in hands-on care. *Nursing Times* 95(27): 48–9.

Clarke M and Stewart J (2000) Handling the wicked issues. In Davies C, Finlay L and Bullman A (eds) *Changing Practice in Health and Social Care.* Open University Press/Sage Publications, London, pp. 377–86.

Collinson D L and Collinson M (1997) 'Delayering Managers': time–space surveillance and its gendered effects. *Organization* 4(3): 375–407.

Cooke J and Standing V (1995) Nurse prescribing. *Pharmaco-economics* 8(4): 271–4.

Cornwall J (1984) *Hard Earned Lives: Accounts of Health and Illness from East London.* Tavistock Publications, London and New York.

Coser R L (1962) *Life in the Ward.* Michigan State University Press, East Lansing.

Cott C (1998) Structure and meaning in multidisciplinary team-work. *Sociology of Health and Illness* 20: 848–71.

Cox C and Baker M (1981) Evaluation: the key to accountability in continuing education. *Journal of Continuing Education in Nursing* 12(1): 11–19.

Coyle J (1999) Exploring the meaning of 'dissatisfaction' with health care: the importance of personal identity threat. *Sociology of Health and Illness* 21(1): 95–124.

Craddock E (1993) Developing the facilitator role in the clinical area. *Nurse Education Today* 13: 217–24.

Crompton R and Sanderson K (1990) *Gendered Jobs and Social Change.* Unwin Hyman, London.

Cunningham G, Dodd T, Grant D, McMurdo M and Richards R (1997) Drug-related problems in elderly patients admitted to Tayside hospitals. *Age and Ageing* 26(5): 375–82.

Darbyshire P (1994) *Living with a Sick Child in Hospital: The Experiences of Parents and Nurses.* Chapman and Hall, London.

Davies C (1995) *Gender and the Professional Predicament in Nursing.* Open University Press, Buckingham.

Davies C and Rosser J (1986) Gendered jobs in the health service: A problem for labour process analysis. In Knights D and Willmott H (eds) *Gender and the Labour Process.* Gower, Aldershot.

Davies K (1989) *Women and Time: Weaving the Strands of Everyday Life.* Grahns Boktryckeri, Lund Sweden.

Davies K (1994) The tensions between process time and clock time in care-work: the example of day nurseries. *Time and Society* 3: 277–304.

Davis D, Thomson M, Oxman A and Haynes R (1992) Evidence for the effectiveness of CME. *JAMA* 268: 1111–17.

Davis D, Thomson M, Oxman A and Haynes R (1995) Changing physician performance. A systematic review of the effect of continuing medical education strategies. *JAMA* 274(9): 700–5.

Davis F (1956) Definitions of time and recovery in paralytic polio convalescence. *American Journal of Sociology* 61: 582–7.

Davis M Z (1980) The organizational, interactional and care-oriented conditions for patient participation in continuity of care: a framework for staff intervention. *Social Science & Medicine* 14A: 39–47.

Daykin N and Clarke B (2000) 'They'll still get the bodily care'. Discourses of care and relationships between nurses and health care assistants in the NHS. *Sociology of Health and Illness* 22(3): 349–64.

De Burgh S, Mant A, Mattick R, Donnelly N, Hall W and Bridges-Webb C (1995) A controlled trial of educational visiting to improve benzodiazepine prescribing in general practice. *Australian Journal of Public Health* 19(2): 142–8.

Deal T and Kennedy A (1982) *Corporate Cultures: The Rites and Rituals of Corporate Life.* Addison Wesley, Cambridge, MA.

Deegan, Mary Jo (1995) The second sex and the Chicago School: women's accounts, knowledge and work. In G A Fine (ed) *A Second Chicago School: The Development of Postwar American Sociology.* University of Chicago Press, Chicago.

Denneby C, Kishi D and Louie C (1996) Drug-related illness in emergency department patients. *American Journal of Health Systems Pharmacy* 53(12): 1422–6.

Department of Health (1989) *Report of the Advisory group on Nurse Prescribing* headed by Crown J. HMSO, London.

Department of Health (1994) *Working in Partnership.* HMSO, London.

Department of Health (1998a) *The New NHS Modern and Dependable: A National Framework for Assessing Performance.* HMSO, London.

Department of Health (1998b) *A First Class Service: Quality in the New NHS.* Department of Health, London.

Department of Health (1999) *Review of Prescribing, Supply and Administration of Medicine.* HMSO, London.

Department of Health (2000a) *A Health Service of all the Talents: Developing the NHS Workforce.* Consultation document on the review of workforce planning. Department of Health. Online. Available: http://www.doh.gov.uk/wfprconsult.

Department of Health (2000b) *Consultation Paper on the Extension of Nurse Prescribing.* HMSO, London.

Department of Health (2001) *Identifying Nurses for Extended Nurse Prescribing Preparation in England.* HMSO, London.

Department of Health and Royal College of Nursing (1994) *Good Practice in the Administration of Depot Neuroleptics: A Guidance Document for Mental Health and Practice Nurses.* HMSO, London.

Department of Health and Social Security (1980) *The Black Report.* HMSO, London.

Department of Health and Social Security (1983) *Inquiry into NHS Management* (The Griffiths Report). Department of Health and Social Security, London.

Department of Trade and Industry (1999) Workers gain new protection from extension of working time directive. Department of Trade and Industry. Online. Available: http://porch.ccta.gov.uk (May 1999).

Devine B A (1978) Nurse–physician interaction: status and social structure within two hospital wards. *Journal of Advanced Nursing* **3**: 287–95.

Dingwall R (1977) *The Social Organisation of Health Visitor Training.* Croom Helm, London.

Dingwall R (1980) Problems of teamwork in primary care. In Lonsdale S, Webb A and Briggs T L (eds) *Teamwork in the Personal Social Services and Health Care.* Croom Helm, London, pp. 111–35.

Dingwall R (1983) In the beginning was the work...reflections on the genesis of occupations. *Sociological Review* **31**: 605–24.

Dingwall R (1996) *Professions and Social Order in a Global Society.* Plenary presentation at ISA Working Group 02 Conference, 11–13 September, University of Nottingham.

Dingwall R and Lewis P (eds) (1983) *The Sociology of the Professions: Lawyers, Doctors and Others.* Macmillan, London.

Dingwall R, Rafferty A M and Webster C (1988) *An Introduction to the Social History of Nursing.* Routledge, London.

Directorate of Nursing and Quality South East Thames Regional Health Authority (1991) *Developing New Roles and Skills for*

Nurses and Midwives. South East Thames Regional Health Authority.

Dowling S (1997) Life can be tough for the inbetweenies. *Nursing Times* **93**(10): 27–8.

Dowling S, Martin R, Skidmore P, Doyal L, Cameron A and Lloyd S (1996) Nurses taking on junior doctors' work: a confusion of accountability. *British Medical Journal* **312**: 1211–14.

Dowswell T, Hewison J and Hinds M (1998) Motivational forces affecting participation in post-registration degree courses and effects on home and work life: a qualitative study. *Journal of Advanced Nursing* **28**: 1326–33.

Dunn E, Bass M, Williams J, Borgiel A, MacDonald P and Spasoff R (1998) Study of the relation of continuing medical education to the quality of family physicians' care. *Journal of Medical Education* **63**(10): 775–84.

Durkheim E (1933) *The Division of Labour in Society.* Collier-MacMillan Ltd, London.

Elliot M A and Turrell A R (1996) Dilemmas for the empowering nurse. *Journal of Nursing Management* **4**: 273–9.

Ersser S J (1997) *Nursing as Therapeutic Activity: An Ethnography.* Avebury, Aldershot.

Etzioni A (ed) (1969) *The Semi-Professions and their Organization: Teachers, Nurses, Social Workers.* Collier-Macmillan, London.

Evans J (1997) Men in nursing: issues of gender segregation and hidden advantage. *Journal of Advanced Nursing* **26**: 226–31.

Ewens A, Howkins E and McClure L (2001) Fit for purpose: does specialist community nurse education prepare nurses for practice? *Nurse Education Today* **21**: 127–35.

Fairhurst E (1977) On being a patient in an orthopaedic ward: some thoughts on the definition of the situation. In Davis A and Horobin G (eds) *Medical Encounters: The Experience of Illness and Treatment.* Croom Helm, London, pp. 159–74.

Fairman J (1992) Watchful vigilance: nursing care, technology, and the development of intensive care units. *Nursing Research* **41**(1): 56–60.

Feiger S M and Schmitt M (1979) Collegiality in interdisciplinary health teams: its measurement and its effects. *Social Science & Medicine* **13**: 217–29.

Ferlie E (1994) The creation and evolution of quasi-markets in the public sector. *Policy and Politics* **222**: 105–12.

Finch F (1990) The politics of community care. In Ungerson C (ed) *Gender and Caring: Work and Welfare in Britain and Scandinavia.* Harvester Wheatsheaf, New York, pp. 34–58.

Firth-Cozens J (1998) Celebrating teamwork. *Quality in Health Care* **S3–S7**, December: 53–7.

Flenniken M (1997) Psychotropic prescriptive patterns among nurse practitioners in nonpsychiatric settings. *Journal of the American Academy of Nurse Practitioners* **9**(3): 117–21.

Fletcher R (1971) *The Making of Sociology: A Study of Sociological Theory. Volume 2, Developments.* Michael Joseph, London.

Flynn R, Williams G and Pickard S (1996) *Markets and Networks: Contracting in Community Health Services.* Open University Press, Buckingham.

Foglesong D, Lambert J and Emerick J (1987) Variables which influence the effect of staff development on nursing practice. *Journal of Continuing Education in Nursing* **18**: 168–71.

Francke A, Garssen B and Huijer Abu-saad H (1995) Determinants of changes in nurses' behaviour after CPE: A literature review. *Journal of Advanced Nursing* **21**: 371–7.

Frankenberg R (1986) Book Review of Cornwall, J. Hard-earned lives: accounts of health and illness from East London. *Sociology of Health and Illness* **8**(1): 99–100.

Frankenberg R (1992) 'Your Time or Mine': temporal contradictions of biomedical practice. In Frankenberg R (ed) *Time, Health and Medicine.* Sage, London, pp. 1–30.

Freidson E (1970a) *Professional Dominance.* Atherton Press Inc., New York.

Freidson E (1970b) *Profession of Medicine: A Study in the Sociology of Applied Knowledge.* Dodd, Mead and Co., New York.

Freidson E (1976) The division of labour as social interaction. *Social Problems* **23**: 304–13.

Friedland R and Boden D (eds) (1994) *NowHere: Time, Space and Modernity.* University of California Press, Berkeley.

Gamarnikow E (1978) Sexual division of labour: the case of nursing. In Kuhn A and Wolpe A M (eds) *Feminism and Materialism.* Routledge and Kegan Paul, London, pp. 96–123.

Gamarnikow E (1991) Nurse or woman? Gender and professionalism in reformed nursing 1860–1923. In Holden P and Littleworth J (eds) *Anthropology and Nursing.* Routledge, London.

Gandhi T, Burstin H, Cook F, Puopolo A, Haas J, Brennan T and Bates D (2000) Drug complications in outpatients. *Journal of General Internal Medicine* **15**: 149–54.

Garfinkel H (1967) *Studies in Ethnomethodology.* Prentice-Hall, New Jersey.

Garvey C, Gross D and Freeman L (1991) Assessing psychotropic medication side effects among children. *Journal of Child & Adolescent Mental Health Nursing* **4**(4): 127–33.

Gilbert A (1995) Nursing: empowerment and the problem of power. *Journal of Advanced Nursing* **16**: 865–71.

Gladstone J (1995) Drug administration errors: a study into the factors underlying the occurrence and reporting of drug errors in a district general hospital. *Journal of Advanced Nursing* **22**: 628–37.

Glaser B and Strauss A L (1965) *Awareness of Dying.* Aldine Publishing Company, Chicago.

Glaser B and Strauss A L (1968) *Time for Dying.* Aldine, Chicago.

Glazer N (1993) *Women's Paid and Unpaid Labor: The Work Transfer in Health Care and Retailing*. Templeton University Press, Philadelphia.

Glennie P and Thrift N (1996) Reworking E. P. Thompson's 'Time, work-discipline and Industrial capitalism'. *Time and Society* **5**(3): 275–99.

Glucksmann M A (1995) Why 'work'? Gender and the 'total social organisation of labour'. *Gender, Work and Organisation* **2**: 63–75.

Glucksmann M A (1998) 'What a difference a day makes': A theoretical and historical exploration of temporality and gender. *Sociology* **32**(2): 239–58.

Goffman E (1959) *The Presentation of Self in Everyday Life*. Doubleday Anchor, New York.

Goffman E (1961) *Asylums: Essays on the Social Situation of Mental Patients and Other Inmates*. Penguin Books, Harmondsworth.

Goffman E (1963) *Stigma: Notes on the Management of Spoiled Identity*. Simon and Schuster, New York.

Goffman E (1971) *Relations in Public: Micro Studies of the Public Order*. Basic Books, New York.

Goffman E (1974) *Frame Analysis: An Essay on the Organization of Experience*. Harper and Row, New York.

Goode D (1994) *A World without Words: The Social Construction of Children Born Deaf and Blind*. Temple University Press, Philadelphia.

Graham H (1985) Providers, negotiators and mediators: women as the hidden carers. In Lewin E and Oelsen V (eds) *Women, Health and Healing: Towards a New Perspective*. Tavistock, London, pp. 25–52.

Gregor F (1997) From women to women: nurses, informal caregivers and the gender dimension of health care reform in Canada. *Health and Social Care in the Community* **5**: 30–6.

Griffiths L (1997) Accomplishing team: teamwork and categorisation in two community mental health teams. *The Sociological Review* **45**: 59–78.

Griffiths L and Hughes D (1994) 'Innocent parties' and 'disheartening' experiences: natural rhetorics in neuro-rehabilitation admissions conferences. *Qualitative Health Research* **4**(4): 385–410.

Griffiths L and Hughes D (2000) Talking contracts and taking care: managers and professionals in the NHS internal market. *Social Science & Medicine* **51**: 209–22.

Gross D (1982) Space, time, and modern culture. *Telos* **50**: 59–78.

Haas J and Shaffir W (1987) *Becoming Doctors: The Adoption of the Cloak of Competence*. JAI Press, London.

Hall E T (1983) *Dance of Life: The Other Dimension of Time*. Anchor Press, Garden, New York.

Hames A and Stirling E (1987) Choice aids recovery. *Nursing Times* **83**(8): 49–51.

Hancock C (1991) Support workers in the UK. *International Nursing Review* **38**(6): 172–6.

Harris C M and Dajda R (1996) The scale of repeat prescribing. *British Journal of General Practice* **46**: 649–53.

Harvath T A, Archbold P G, Stewart B J, Godow S, Kirshling J M, Miller L L, Hogan J, Brody K and Schook J (1994) Establishing partnerships with family caregivers: local and cosmopolitan knowledge. *Journal of Gerontological Nursing* **20**: 29–35.

Health Services Management Unit (1996) *The Future Health Care Workforce: The Steering Group Report*. Health Services Management Unit, University of Manchester.

Hefferin E A (1979) Health goal setting: Patient–nurse collaboration at VA facilities. *Military Medicine* December: 814–22.

Helman C (1992) Heart disease and the cultural construction of time. In Frankenberg R (ed) *Time, Health and Medicine*. Sage, London, pp. 31–55.

Henley N (1977) *Body Politics: Power, Sex and Nonverbal Communication*. Prentice-Hall, Englewood Cliffs, NJ.

Heslop L, McIntyre M and Ives G (2001) Undergraduate student nurses' expectations and their self-reported preparedness for the graduate year role. *Journal of Advanced Nursing* **36**(5): 626–34.

Hewison A and Wildman S (1996) The theory/practice gap in nursing: a new dimension. *Journal of Advanced Nursing* **24**: 754–61.

Hochschild A (1989) *The Second Shift: Working Parents and the Revolution at Home*. Judy Piatkus, London.

Hokenstad M C and Johansson L (1990) Caregivers for the elderly in Sweden: program challenges and policy initiatives. In Biegel D E and Blum A (eds) *Aging and Care-giving: Theory, Research, and Policy*. Sage, Newberry Park, CA, pp. 254–69.

Hood C (1991) A public management for all seasons. *Public Administration* **69**(1): 3–19.

Howie J, Heaney D and Maxwell M (1994) Evaluating care of patients reporting pain in fundholding practices. *British Medical Journal* **309**: 705–10.

Hughes D (1988) When nurse knows best: some aspects of nurse–doctor interaction in a casualty department. *Sociology of Health and Illness* **10**: 1–22.

Hughes D (1996) NHS managers as rhetoricians: a case of culture management? *Sociology of Health and Illness* **18**: 291–314.

Hughes D and Allen D (1993a) *Inside the Black Box: Obstacles to Change in the Modern Hospital*. Final report submitted to the King's Fund and Milbank Memorial Fund: Joint Health Policy Review.

Hughes D and Allen D (1993b) *Expanded Nursing Roles, Junior Doctors' Hours and the Hospital Division of Labour: A Pilot Study*. Final Report for South East Thames Regional Health Authority.

Hughes E C (1958) *Men and Their Work*. The Free Press, Glencoe, Illinois.

Hughes E C (1984) *The Sociological Eye.* Transaction Books, New Brunswick and London.

Hutton C (1987) Impact of mandatory continuing education: a review of research on nurses' attitudes and perceived outcomes. *Journal of Continuing Education in Nursing* 18(6): 209–13.

Illich I (1976) *Medical Nemesis: The Expropriation of Health.* Marion Boyars, London.

Jacono B and Jacono J (1994) Power tactics and their potential impact on nursing. *Journal of Advanced Nursing* 19: 954–9.

James N (1992a) Care = organisation + physical labour + emotional labour. *Sociology of Health and Illness* 14: 488–509.

James N (1992b) Care, work and carework: a synthesis? In Robinson J, Gray A and Elkan R (eds) *Policy Issues in Nursing.* Open University Press, Milton-Keynes.

Jamous H and Peloille B (1970) Changes in the French university-hospital system. In Jackson J A (ed) *Professions and Professionalization.* Cambridge University Press, Cambridge, pp. 111–52.

Jewell S E (1994) Patient participation: what does it mean to nurses? *Journal of Advanced Nursing* 19: 433–8.

Johnson T J (1967) *Professions and Power.* Macmillan, London.

Jordan S (1998) From classroom theory to clinical practice: evaluating the impact of a post-registration course. *Nurse Education Today* 18(4): 293–302.

Jordan S and Hughes D (1998) Using bioscience knowledge in nursing: actions, interactions and reactions. *Journal of Advanced Nursing* 27(5): 1060–8.

Jordan S and Hughes D (2000) Community teamwork is key to monitoring the side effects of medication. *Nursing Times/BMJ inaugural joint issue* 96(15): 39–40.

Jordan S and Reid K (1997) The biological sciences in nursing: an empirical paper reporting on the applications of physiology to nursing care. *Journal of Advanced Nursing* 26(1): 169–79.

Jordan S, Coleman M, Hardy B and Hughes D (1999) Assessing educational effectiveness: the impact of a specialist course on the delivery of care. *Journal of Advanced Nursing* 30(4): 796–807.

Jordan S (1998) From classroom theory to clinical practice: evaluating the impact of a post-registration course. *Nurse Education Today* 18(4): 293–302.

Kanouse D and Jacoby I (1988) When does information change practitioners' behaviour? *International Journal of Technology Assessment in Health Care* 4: 27–33.

Keddy B, Gillis M J, Jacobs P, Burton H and Rogers M (1986) The doctor–nurse relationship: an historical perspective. *Journal of Advanced Nursing* 11(6): 745–53.

Kelly B (1996) Hospital Nursing: 'Its a battle!' A follow up study of English graduate nurses. *Journal of Advanced Nursing* 24: 1063–9.

Kennedy I (2001) *Learning from Bristol: The Report of the Public Inquiry into Children's Heart Surgery at the Bristol Royal Infirmary 1984–1995*. HMSO, Norwich.

Kitson A (1987) A comparative analysis of lay-caring and professional (nursing) caring relationships. *International Journal of Nursing Studies* 24: 155–65.

Knaus W A, Draper E A, Wagner D P and Zimmerman J E (1986) An evaluation of outcome from intensive care in major medical centres. *Annals of Internal Medicine* 104: 410–18.

Kohn L, Corrigan J and Donaldson M (2000) *To Err is Human: Building a Safer Health System*. National Academy Press, Washington DC.

Kristiansen I and Holtedahl K (1993) Effect of remuneration system on the general practitioner's choice between surgery consultations and home visits. *Journal of Epidemiology and Community Health* 47: 481–4.

Kushlick A (1976) Evidence to the Committee of Inquiry into Mental Handicap Nursing and Care (The Jay Committee) HCERT Research Report 120, Wessex Regional Health Authority, Winchester.

Land L, Mhaolrunaigh S and Castledine G (1996) Effect and effectiveness of the scope of professional practice. *Nursing Times* 92(35): 32–5.

Larkin G V (1983) *Occupational Monopoly and Modern Medicine*. Tavistock, London.

Larson E (1999) The impact of physician–nurse interaction on patient care. *Holistic Nursing* 13: 38–47.

Larson M (1977) *The Rise of Professionalism*. University of California Press, Berkeley.

Latimer J (2000) *The Conduct of Care: Understanding Nursing Practice*. Blackwell Science, Oxford.

Lave J (1988a) *Cognition in Practice: Mind Mathematics and Culture in Everyday Life*. Cambridge University Press, New York.

Lave J (1988b) *The Culture of Acquisition and the Practice of Understanding*. Report No. IRL 88-0007. Institute for Research and Learning, Palo Alto, CA

Lawler J (1991) *Behind the Screens: Nursing, Somology and the Problem of the Body*. Churchill Livingstone, London.

Lemp H (1995) Nursing: no regrets. *British Medical Journal* 311: 307–8.

Levy J A (1982) The staging of negotiations between hospice and medical institutions. *Urban Life* 11(3): 293–311.

Lewis J and Meredith B (1988) *Daughters who Care: Daughters Caring for Mothers at Home*. Routledge and Kegan Paul, London.

Liaschenko J (1994) The moral geography of home care. *Advanced Nursing Science* 17(2): 16–26.

Lief H I and Fox R C (1963) Training for 'detached concern' in medical students. In Lief H, Lief V F, Lief N R (eds) *The Psychological Basis of Medical Practice*, pp. 12–35.

Light D (1975) The sociological calendar: an analytical tool for fieldwork applied to medical and psychiatric training. *American Journal of Sociology* **80**: 1145–64.

Lindley C, Tulley M, Paramsothy V and Tallis R (1992) Inappropriate medication is a major cause of adverse drug reactions in elderly patients. *Age and Ageing* **21**: 294–300.

Luker K, Austin L, Hogg C, Willock J, Wright K, Ferguson B, Clark S J and Smith K (1997) *Evaluation of Nursing Prescribing: Final Report.* University of Liverpool.

MacIntyre S and Oldman D (1977) Coping with migraine. In Davis A and Horobin G (eds) *Medical Encounters: The Experience of Illness and Treatment.* Croom Helm, London, pp. 55–71.

Mackay L (1993) *Conflicts in Care. Medicine and Nursing.* Chapman and Hall, London.

MacPherson K I (1991) Looking at caring and nursing through a feminist lens. In Neil R M and Watts R (eds) *Caring and Nursing: Explorations in Feminist Perspectives.* National League for Nursing, New York, pp. 25–42.

Macy B A and Izumi H (1993) Organizational change, design and work innovation: a meta-analysis of 131 North American field studies 1961–91. In Pasmore W A and Woodman R W (eds) *Research in Organizational Change and Development.* Vol. 7. Greenwich, CT: JAI Press, pp. 235–313.

Malin N and Teasdale K (1991) Caring versus empowerment: considerations for nursing practice. *Journal of Advanced Nursing* **16**: 657–62.

Malmberg B (1995) Problems of time–space co-ordination: a key to the understanding of multiplant firms. *Progress in Human Geography* **19**(1): 47–60.

Marx K (1970 [1887]) *Capital* (Vol. 1). Lawrence and Wishart, London.

Mauksch H O (1965) The nurse, coordinator of patient care. In Skipper J K and Leonard R R (eds) *Social Interaction and Patient Care.* JB Lippincott Company, Philadelphia, pp. 251–66.

Mauksch H O (1966) The organizational context of nursing practice. In Davis F (ed) *The Nursing Profession: Five Sociological Essays.* Wiley, New York, pp. 109–37.

Mauksch H O (1966) The organizational context of nursing practice. In Davis F (ed) *The Nursing Profession: Five Sociological Essays.* John Wiley and Sons Inc, New York, pp. 109–38.

May C (1992) Nursing work, nurses' knowledge, and the subjectification of the patient. *Sociology of Health and Illness* **14**(4): 472–87.

McClosky J (1981) The effects of nursing education on job effectiveness: an overview of the literature. *Research in Nursing & Health* **4**: 355–73.

McIntosh J (1977) *Communication and Awareness in a Cancer Ward.* Croom Helm, London.

Mead D and McGuire J (1993) *Innovations in Nursing Practice: The Development of Primary Nursing in Wales*. NHS Wales.

Mechanic D (1961) Sources of power of lower participants in complex organizations. *Administrative Science Quarterly* 7: 349–64.

Medicines Control Agency (2001) *Extended Prescribing of Prescription only Medicines by Independent Nurse Prescribers*. Medicines Control Agency, London.

Meehan A J (1981) Some conversational features in the use of medical terms by doctors and patients. In Atkinson P and Heath C (eds) *Medical Work: Realities and Routines*. Gower, Westmead, pp. 107–27.

Meerabeau L (1998) Project 2000 and the nature of nursing knowledge. In Abbott P and Meerabeau L (eds) (2nd edn) *The Sociology of the Caring Professions*. UCL Press, London, pp. 82–105.

Melia K (1983) Becoming and being a nurse. In Thompson I, Melia K and Boyd K (eds) *Nursing Ethics*. Churchill Livingstone, Edinburgh, pp. 14–33.

Melia K M (1979) A sociological approach to the analysis of nursing work. *Journal of Advanced Nursing* 4: 57–67.

Melia K M (1987) *Learning and Working: The Occupational Socialization of Nurses*. Tavistock, London.

Menzies I (1963) A case study in the functioning of social systems as a defence against anxiety: a report on a study of the nursing service of a general hospital. *Human Relations* 13: 95–121.

Meservy D and Monson M (1987) Impact of continuing education on nursing practice and quality of patient care. *Journal of Continuing Education in Nursing* 18(6): 214–20.

Meyer J (1993) Lay participation in care: a challenge for multidisciplinary teamwork. *Journal of Interprofessional Care* 7(1): 57–66.

Miers M (2000) *Gender Issues and Nursing Practice*. Macmillan, London.

Miller J (1995) The adverse drug reaction: a clinical opportunity for pharmacists. *Hospital Pharmacy* 30: 769–73.

Millman M (1976) *The Unkindest Cut: Life in the Backrooms of Medicine*. William Morrow and Company, Inc., New York.

Montenko A K (1988) Respite care and pride in caregiving: the experience of six older men caring for their disabled wives. In Reinharz S and Rowles G (eds) *Qualitative Gerontology*. Springer, New York, pp. 104–27.

Moore W E (1963) *Man, Time and Society*. John Wiley and Sons Inc., New York and London.

Moores Y (1992) Scope for extensions. *Nursing Times* 88(37): 28–9.

Mueller M R (1997) Science versus care: physicians, nurses and the dilemma of clinical research. In Elston M A (ed) *The Sociology of Medical Science and Technology*. Blackwell, Oxford, pp. 57–78.

Mumford E (1970) *Interns: From Students to Physicians*. Harvard University Press, Cambridge, Massachusetts.

Myers L C (1979) *The Socialization of Neophyte Nurses.* UMI Research Press, Michigan.

National Health Service Management Executive (1991) *Junior Doctors: The New Deal.* National Health Service Management Executive, London.

Needleman R and Nelson A (1988) Policy implications: the worth of women's work. In Stratham A, Miller E and Mauksch H (eds) *The Worth of Women's Work: A Qualitative Synthesis.* State University of New York, New York, pp. 293–307.

NHS (2000) *The NHS Plan. A Plan for Investment. A Plan for Reform.* Cmnd 4818-I, Norwich, HMSO. Online. Available: http://www.nhs.uk/nhs/plan.

Nolan M, Grant G and Keady J (1996) *Understanding Family Care.* Open University Press, Buckingham.

Nolan M, Owens R G and Nolan J (1995) Continuing professional education: identifying the characteristics of an effective system. *Journal of Advanced Nursing* 21: 551–60.

Oakley A (1974a) *Housewife.* Penguin Books, London.

Oakley A (1974b) *The Sociology of Housework.* Martin Robertson, Oxford.

Oakley A (1984) The importance of being a nurse. *Nursing Times* 80(50): 24–7.

Ogier M E (1989) *Working and Learning.* Scutari Press, London.

Orem D E (1995) *Nursing: Concepts of Practice (5th edition).* Mosby, St Louis.

Ovretveit J, Mathias P and Thompson T (1997) *Interprofessional Relations.* Macmillan, Basingstoke.

Oxman A D (1994) *No Magic Bullets.* North East Regional Health Authority, London.

Parsons T (1951) *The Social System.* Routledge and Kegan Paul, London.

Paton C (1993) Devolution and centralism in the National Health Service. *Social Policy and Administration* 27(2): 83–108.

Perry L (1995) Continuing professional education: luxury or necessity? *Journal of Advanced Nursing* 21: 766–71.

Peters T J and Waterman R H (1982) *In Search of Excellence: Lessons From America's Best-Run Companies.* Harper and Row, New York.

Phillips A and Taylor B (1980) Sex and skill: notes towards a feminist economics. *Feminist Review* 6: 79–88.

Pilnick A (1998) 'Why didn't you just say that?' Dealing with issues of asymmetry, knowledge and competence in the pharmacist/client encounter. *Sociology of Health and Illness* 20(1): 29–51.

Pirmohamed M, Breckenridge A, Kitteringham N and Park B K (1998) Adverse drug reactions. *British Medical Journal* 316: 1295–8.

Porter S (1991) A participant observation study of power relations between nurses and doctors in a general hospital. *Journal of Advanced Nursing* 16: 728–35.

Porter S (1995) *Nursing's Relationship with Medicine: A Critical Realist Ethnography.* Avebury, Aldershot.

Pouyanne P, Haramburu F, Imbs J and Begaud B (2000) Admissions to hospital caused by adverse drug reactions: cross sectional incidence study. *British Medical Journal* 320: 1036.

Pritchard P (1992) Doctors, patients and time. In Frankenberg R (ed) *Time, Health and Medicine.* Sage, London, pp. 75–93.

Proctor S (1989) The functioning of nursing routines in the management of a transient work force. *Journal of Advanced Nursing* 14: 180–9.

Prowse M A and Lyne P A (2000a) Revealing the contribution of bioscience-based nursing knowledge to clinically effective care. *Clinical Effectiveness in Nursing* 4(2): 67–75.

Prowse M A and Lyne PA (2000b) Clinical effectiveness in the postanaesthesia care unit; the development of knowledge which contributes to achieving intended patient outcomes. *Journal of Advanced Nursing* 30(5): 1115–24.

Purkis M E (1996) Nursing in quality space: technologies governing experiences of care. *Nursing Inquiry* 3(2): 101–11.

Quint J C (1972) Institutionalised practices of information control. In Freidson E and Lorber J (eds) *Medical Men and Their Work.* Aldine Atherton, Inc., Chicago, pp. 220–38.

Qureshi H (1990) Boundaries between formal and informal caregiving work. In Ungerson C (ed) *Gender and Caring: Work and Welfare in Britain and Scandinavia.* Harvester Wheatsheaf, London, pp. 59–79.

Radley A and Billig M (1996) Accounts of health and illness: dilemmas and representation. *Sociology of Health and Illness* 18(2): 220–40.

Rafferty A M (1996) *The Politics of Nursing Knowledge.* Routledge, London.

Rafferty A M, Allock N and Lathean J (1996) The theory/practice gap: taking issue with the issue. *Journal of Advanced Nursing* 23: 685–91.

Ranade W (1994) *A Future for the NHS? Health Care in the 1990s.* Longman, London and New York.

Rittenhouse B (1994) Economic incentives and disincentives for efficient prescribing. *Pharmacoeconomics* 6(3): 222–32.

Robinson M (1994) Evaluation of medical audit. *Journal of Epidemiology & Community Health* 48: 435–40.

Rochon B and Gurwitz J (1997) Optimising drug treatment for elderly people: the prescribing cascade. *BMJ* 315: 1096–9.

Rokstad K and Straand J (1997) Drug prescribing during direct and indirect contacts with patients in general practice. *Scandinavian Journal of Primary Health Care* 15(2): 103–8.

Rose H and Bruce E (1995) Mutual care but differential esteem: caring between older couples. In Arber S and Ginn J (eds)

Connecting Gender and Ageing: A Sociological Approach. Open University Press, Buckingham, pp. 114–28.

Rosengren W and Devault S (1963) The sociology of time and space in an obstetrical hospital. In Freidson E (ed) *The Hospital in Modern Society*. Free Press, New York, pp. 266–91.

Rosenthal C, Marshall V W, MacPherson A S and French S E (1980) *Nurses, Patients and Families*. Croom Helm, London.

Ross F (1987) *Evaluation of a Drug Guide in Primary Care*. Unpublished PhD thesis, University of London.

Roth J (1963) *Timetables: Structuring the Passage of Time in Hospital and other Careers*. The Bobbs-Merrill Company Inc., New York.

Roth J and Douglas D (1983) *No Appointment Necessary: The Hospital Emergency Department in the Medical Services World*. Irving Publishers, New York.

Roughead E, Gilbert A, Primrose J and Samson L (1998) Drug-related hospital admissions, a review of Australian studies published 1988–96. *Medical Journal of Australia* 168: 405–8.

Rowe H (1996) Multidisciplinary teamwork – myth or reality. *Journal of Nursing Management* 4: 93–101.

Royal College of General Practitioners (1985) *What Sort of Doctor?: Assessing Quality of Care in General Practice*. Report from general practice no.23. Royal College of General Practitioners, London.

Rufli G M (1996) Changing roles for psychiatric clinical nurse specialists: prescriptive privileges. *Kentucky Nurse* 44(4): 16–17.

Rupp M (1992) Value of community pharmacists' interventions to correct prescribing errors. *Annals of Pharmacotherapeutics* 26(12): 1580–4.

Rushing W A (1965) Social influence and the social psychological function of deference: a study of psychiatric nursing. In Skipper J K and Leonard R C (eds) *Social Interaction and Patient Care*. Blackwell Scientific Publications, Oxford and Edinburgh, pp. 366–76.

Ryan A (1996) Doctor–nurse relations: a review of the literature. *Social Sciences in Health* 2(2): 93–106.

Salvage J (1988) Partnerships in care? An exploration of the theory and practice of the new nursing in the UK. Unpublished M.Sc. dissertation, Royal Holloway and Bedford New College, University of London.

Salvage J (1992) The new nursing: empowering patients or empowering nurses? In Robinson J, Gray A and Elkan R (eds) *Policy Issues in Nursing*. Open University Press, Milton Keynes, pp. 9–23.

Savage J (1987) *Nurses, Gender and Sexuality*. Heinemann Nursing, London.

Savage J (1995) *Nursing Intimacy: An Ethnographic Approach to Nurse–Patient Interaction*. Scutari Press, London.

Scheff T J (1961) Control over policy by attendants in a mental hospital. *Journal of Health and Human Behaviour* 2: 93–105.

Scheller M (1993) A qualitative analysis of factors in the work environment that influence nurses' use of knowledge gained from CE programs. *Journal of Continuing Education in Nursing* **24**: 114–22.

Schneider P, Gift M, Lee Y, Rothermich A and Sill B (1995) Cost of medication-related problems at a university hospital. *American Journal of Health-System Pharmacy* **52**: 2415–8.

Schwartz B (1979) Waiting, exchange, and power: the distribution of time in social systems. In Robboy H, Greenblatt S L and Clark C (eds) *Social Interaction: Introductory Readings in Sociology.* St Martin's Press, New York, pp. 240–65.

Silverman D (1993) *Interpreting Qualitative Data. Methods for Analyzing Talk, Text and Interaction.* Sage, London.

Smith A (1976 [1776]) *An Inquiry into the Nature and Causes of the Wealth of Nations* (Vol. 1). Clarendon Press, Oxford.

Smith M (1991) (2nd edn) *Fluids and Electrolytes.* Churchill Livingstone, Edinburgh.

Snelgrove S and Hughes D (2000) Interprofessional relations between doctors and nurses: perspectives from South Wales. *Journal of Advanced Nursing* **31**: 661–7.

Spitzer W, Sackett D, Sibley J, Roberts R, Gent M, Kergin D, Hackett B and Olynich A (1974) The Burlington Randomised trial of the nurse practitioner. *New England Journal of Medicine* **290**: 251–6.

Stacey M (1988) *The Sociology of Health and Healing.* Unwin Hyman, London.

Stacey M (1992) *Regulating British Medicine: The General Medical Council.* Wiley, Chichester.

Starkey K (1992) Time and the hospital consultant. In Frankenberg R (ed) *Time, Health and Medicine.* Sage, London, pp. 94–107.

Stein L I (1967) The doctor–nurse game. *Archives of General Psychiatry* **16**: 699–703.

Stein L I, Watts D T and Howell T (1990) The doctor–nurse game revisited. *Nursing Outlook* **36**(6): 264–8.

Stelfox H T, Chua G, O'Rourke K and Detsky A (1998) Conflict of interest in the debate over calcium channel antagonists. *New England Journal of Medicine* **338**(2): 101–6.

Stevens R and Balon D (1997) Detection of hazardous drug/drug interactions in a community pharmacy and subsequent intervention. *International Journal of Pharmacy Practice* **5**: 142–8.

Stockley I (1999) *Drug Interactions (5th edition).* Pharmaceutical Press, London.

Strauss A L (1978) *Negotiations: Varieties, Contexts, Processes and Social Order.* Jossey-Bass, London.

Strauss A L, Fagerhaugh S, Suczek B and Wiener C (1982a) The work of hospitalised patients. *Social Science & Medicine* **16**: 977–86.

Strauss A L, Fagerhaugh S, Suczek B and Wiener C (1982b) Sentimental work in the technologized hospital. *Sociology of Health and Illness* **4**: 254–77.

Strauss A L, Fagerhaugh S, Suczek B and Wiener C (1985) *The Social Organization of Medical Work*. University of Chicago Press, Chicago.

Strauss A, Schatzman L, Bucher R, Ehrlich D and Sabshin M (1963) The hospital and its negotiated order. In Freidson E (ed) *The Hospital in Modern Society*. Free Press, New York, pp. 147–69.

Strauss A, Schatzman L, Bucher R, Ehrlich D and Sabshin M (1964) *Psychiatric Ideologies and Institutions*. The Free Press of Glencoe Collier-Macmillan Limited, London.

Strong P M and Robinson J (1990) *The NHS: Under New Management*. Open University Press, Buckingham.

Strong P M (1979) *The Ceremonial Order of the Clinic*. Routledge and Kegan Paul, London.

Sudnow D (1967) *Passing On*. Prentice-Hall, Inc., Englewood Cliffs, New Jersey.

Sugrue N M (1982) Emotions as property and context for negotiation. *Urban Life* **11**(3): 280–92.

Sulch D and Kalra L (2000) Integrated care pathways in stroke management. *Age and Ageing* **29**(4): 349–52.

Sullivan O (1997) Time waits for no (wo)man: an investigation of the gendered experience of domestic time. *Sociology* **31**(2): 221–39.

Svensson R (1996) The interplay between doctors and nurses – a negotiated order perspective. *Sociology of Health and Illness* **18**(3): 379–98.

Taraborrelli P (1994) Innocents, converts and oldhands: the experiences of Alzheimer's disease caregivers. In Bloor M and Taraborrelli P (eds) *Qualitative Studies in Health and Medicine*. Aldershot, Avebury, pp. 22–42.

Taylor C (1970) *In Horizontal Orbit: Hospitals and the Cult of Efficiency*. Holt, Rhinehart and Whinston, USA.

Taylor M J (1975) Organisational growth, spatial interaction and location. *Regional Studies* **13**: 421–37.

Tellis-Nayak M and Tellis-Nayak V (1984) Games that professionals play: the social psychology of physician–nurse interactions. *Social Science & Medicine* **18**(12): 1063–9.

Tempkin-Greener H (1983) Interprofessional perspectives on teamwork in health care: a care study. *Milbank Memorial Fund Quarterly* **61**: 641–58.

Thompson E (1967) Time, work-discipline, and industrial capitalism. *Past and Present* **38**: 56–97.

Tierney L (1995) Blood vessels and lymphatics. In Tierney L M, McPhee S J and Papadakis M (eds) *Current Medical Diagnosis and Treatment*. Lange Medical, Prentice Hall, London, pp. 391–422.

Timmermans S (1999) *Sudden Death and the Myth of CPR.* Temple University Press, Philadelphia.

Towell D (1975) *Understanding Psychiatric Nursing.* Royal College of Nursing, London.

Trnobranski P (1994) Nurse–patient negotiation: assumption or reality. *Journal of Advanced Nursing* 19: 733–7.

Twigg J and Atkin K (1994) *Carers Perceived: Policy and Practice in Informal Care.* Open University Press, Buckingham.

UKCC (1987) *Project 2000: The Final Proposals.* UKCC, London.

UKCC (1992) *The Scope of Professional Practice.* UKCC, London.

UKCC (1999a) *A Higher Level of Practice: Draft Descriptor and Standard.* UKCC.

UKCC (1999b) A Higher Level of Practice: The UKCC's Proposals for Recognising a Higher Level of Practice within the Post Registration Regulatory Framework, UKCC. Online. Available: http://www.ukcc.org.uk/A%20higher%20level%of%20practice.htm.

Ungerson C (1983) Women and caring: skills, tasks and taboos. In Gamarnikow E, Morgan D, Purvis J and Taylorson D (eds) *The Public and the Private.* Heinemann, London, pp. 62–77.

Ungerson C (1990) The language of care: crossing the boundaries. In Ungerson C (ed) *Gender and Caring: Work and Welfare in Britain and Scandinavia.* Harvester Wheatsheaf, London, pp. 8–33.

US Office of Technology Assessment (1986) *Nurse Practitioners, Physicians' Assistants And Certified Nurse-Midwives; Policy Analysis.* US Government Printing Office, Washington DC.

Waddell D (1991) The effects of continuing education on nursing practice: a meta-analysis. *Journal of Continuing Education in Nursing* 22(3): 113–18.

Wade S (1995) Partnership in care: a critical review. *Nursing Standard* 9(48): 29–30, 32.

Walby S (1989) Flexibility and the changing sexual division of labour. In Woods S (ed) *The Transformation of Work.* Unwin Hyman, London.

Walby S and Greenwell J with Mackay L and Soothill K (1994) *Medicine and Nursing: Professions in a Changing Health Service.* Sage, London.

Wallace H and Solomon J (1999) Quality of epilepsy treatment and services: the views of women with epilepsy. *Seizure* 8: 81–7.

Waterworth S and Luker K (1990) Reluctant collaborators: do patients want to be involved in decisions concerning their care? *Journal of Advanced Nursing* 15: 971–6.

Webb B (1977) Trauma and tedium: an account of living on a children's ward. In Davis A and Horobin G (eds) *Medical Encounters: The Experience of Illness and Treatment.* Croom Helm, London, pp. 175–90.

Wessen A F (1958) Hospital ideology and communication between ward personnel. In Jaco E G (ed) (1st edn) *Patients, Physicians and Illness.* Free Press, Glencoe, Illinois, pp. 448–68.

Wicks D (1998) *Nurses and Doctors at Work: Rethinking Professional Boundaries.* Open University Press, Buckingham.

Wilson H S (1993) Family care-giving for a relative with Alzheimer's dementia: coping with negative choices. In Wegner G and Alexander R (eds) *Readings in Family Nursing.* Philadelphia: JB Lippincott, pp. 197–207.

Wilson R N (1958) Team work in the operating room. In Jaco E G (ed) (1st edn) *Patients, Physicians and Illness: Sourcebook in Behavioral Science and Medicine.* Free Press, Glencoe, Illinois, pp. 491–501.

Witz A (1986) Patriarchy and the labour market: occupational control strategies and the medical division of labour. In Knights D and Willmott H (eds) *Gender and the Labour Process.* Gower, Hampshire, pp. 14–53.

Witz A (1988) Patriarchal relations and patterns of sex segregation in the medical division of labour. In Walby S (ed) *Gender Segregation at Work.* Open University Press, Milton Keynes, pp. 74–90.

Witz A (1992) *Professions and Patriarchy.* Routledge, London.

Witz A (1994) The challenge of nursing. In Gabe J, Kelleher D and Williams G (eds) *Challenging Medicine.* Routledge, London, pp. 23–45.

Wolf Z R (1988) *Nurses' Work: The Sacred and the Profane.* University of Pennsylvania Press, Philadelphia.

Wright M and Parker G (1998) Incident monitoring in psychiatry. *Journal of Quality Clinical Practice* **18**: 249–61.

Wright S (1995) The role of the nurse: extended or expanded? *Nursing Standard* **9**(33): 25–9.

Zarit S H, Pearlin L I and Warner Schaie K (1993) *Caregiving Systems: Informal and Formal Helpers.* Hillsdale, New Jersey: Lawrence Erlbaum Associates, Publishers.

Zermansky A (1996) Who controls repeats? *British Journal of General Practice* **46**(412): 643–7.

Zerubavel E (1979a) *Patterns of Time in Hospital Life.* Chicago University Press, Chicago.

Zerubavel E (1979b) The temporal organization of continuity: the case of medical and nursing coverage. *Human Organization* **38**(1): 78–83.

Zussman R (1992) *Intensive Care.* University of Chicago Press, Chicago.

Zwarenstein M and Reeves S (2000) What's so great about collaboration? *British Medical Journal* **320**: 1022–3.

Index of names

Abbott A   16, 18,
  102–3, 106, 109
Adam B   44
Allan H   158, 159,
  164, 177, 208
Allen D   5, 84
Anspach R R   42
Avis M   156

Benner P E   85
Brooking J   162,
  208
Bury M   154

Campbell-Heider N
  73
Caress A L   157
Cornwall J   69
Cott C   71
Coyle J   158, 159,
  164

Darbyshire P   157
Davies C   8, 9, 31,
  44
Davis M Z   172
Devault S   80
Dingwall R   15, 16,
  72, 157
Durkheim E   3,
  10–13, 14

Elliott M A   170
Ersser S J   157

Fairman   138
Frankenberg R   27,
  28, 29, 44
Freidson E   3, 4, 8,
  77, 153

Garfinkel H   164
Glaser B G   185,
  203
Glennie P   26
Goffman E   164
Greenwell J   39,
  138

Hall E T   25, 30,
  31
Harvath T A   192
Hughes D   78, 79,
  89
Hughes E C
  13–15, 18, 80,
  81, 101–2, 105,
  106, 114,
  160–1, 191,
  192, 193

James N   199, 200
Jamous H   106
Johnson T J   153

Kennedy I   56
Kushlick A   44

Larkin G   4, 5, 6
Larson E   74
Larson M   153
Lawler J   96, 194,
  199

Mauksch H O   42,
  47
Meehan H   167

Nolan M   192

Orem D E   168

Oxman A D   130

Parsons T   152, 153
Peloille B   106
Pilnick A   167
Pollock D   73
Porter S   78, 79

Rosengren W   80
Rosenthal   185, 187,
  188, 203, 204
Roth J A   165
Rushing W A   77

Salvage J   105, 157
Savage J   179
Stein L I   5, 75, 77,
  78, 79, 81, 89,
  91
Stockley I   142
Strauss A L   37,
  164, 172, 179,
  185, 203, 204
Svensson R   5, 62,
  84

Tellis-Nayak M   79,
  80
Tellis-Nayak V   79,
  80
Thrift N   26
Timmermans S   96
Trnobranski P   156
Turrell A R   170

Walby S   39, 138
Webb C   170
Wilson R N   80

Zerubavel E   37

Subject index